ABC OF ASTHMA

ABC OF ASTHMA

Fourth edition

JOHN REES

Senior Lecturer and Consultant Physician,
Guy's and St Thomas' Hospitals, London

DIPAK KANABAR

Consultant Paediatrician,
Guy's and St Thomas' Hospitals, London

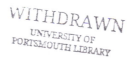
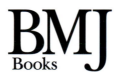
BMJ
Books

© BMJ Books 2000
BMJ Books is an imprint of the BMJ Publishing Group
BMA House, Tavistock Square, London WC1H 9JR
www.bmjbooks.com

First published 1984
by the BMJ Publishing Group,
Second edition 1984
Reprinted 1991, 1992
Third edition 1995
Reprinted 1996, 1997
Fourth edition 2000

British Library Cataloguing in Publication Data

A catalogue record for this book is available from the British Library

ISBN 0-7279-1261-5

Editorial production by WordWise, Lee-on-the-Solent, Hampshire
Typeset by Phoenix Photosetting, Chatham, Kent
Colour origination by Tenon and Polert, Hong Kong
Printed and bound in China

CONTENTS

ASTHMA IN ADULTS – John Rees

1. Definition and pathology 1
2. Prevalence 4
3. Diagnostic testing and monitoring 7
4. Clinical course 12
5. Precipitating factors 16
6. General management of acute asthma 23
7. Treatment of acute asthma 26
8. General management of chronic asthma 32
9. Treatment of chronic asthma 35
10. Methods of delivering drugs 42

ASTHMA IN CHILDREN – Dipak Kanabar

11. Definition, prevalence and prevention 45
12. Patterns of illness and diagnosis 50
13. Treatment 54
14. Drug treatment 55
15. Acute severe asthma 62
Index 64

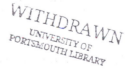

Abbreviations

ACTH	adrenocorticotropic hormone
BTS	British Thoracic Society
CFC	chlorofluocarbon
COPD	chronic obstructive pulmonary disease
FEV_1	forced expiratory volume in 1 second
IGF1	insulin-like growth factor-1
ISAAC	International Study of Asthma and Allergies in Childhood
MDI	metered dose inhaler
NHLBI	National Heart, Lung and Blood Institute (United States)
PEF	peak expiratory flow
PEFR	peak expiratory flow rate

1 Definition and pathology

Asthma is a common condition, which seems to be increasing in prevalence in most studies around the world. The prevalence depends on the diagnosis used and the population studied. Moderately severe asthma with attacks of wheezing that are precipitated by specific stimuli is relatively easy to recognise. There may be difficulties with more severe disease when lung function never returns completely to normal between attacks, particularly in older people. In mild cases obstruction of airflow may be intermittent with no symptoms of asthma between events.

The clinical characteristic of asthma is airflow obstruction, which can be reversed over short periods of time or with treatment. This may be evident from provocation by specific stimuli or from the response to bronchodilator drugs. The airflow obstruction leads to the usual symptoms of shortness of breath. The underlying pathology is inflammatory change in the airway wall leading to irritability and responsiveness to various stimuli – and also to coughing, the other common symptom of asthma.

Asthma has commonly been defined on the basis of wide variations over short periods of time in resistance to airflow. Recent definitions have come to recognise the importance of the inflammatory change in the airways.

Low concentrations of non-specific stimuli such as inhaled methacholine and histamine produce a reaction from the inflamed airway. In general, the more severe the asthma the greater the inflammation and the more the airways react on challenge. Other stimuli such as cold air, exercise, and hypotonic solutions can also provoke this increased reactivity. In contrast, it is difficult to induce significant narrowing of the airways with many of these stimuli in healthy people. In some epidemiological studies increased airway responsiveness is used as part of the definition of asthma. Wheezing during the past 12 months is added to exclude those who have increased responsiveness but no symptoms.

In clinical practice in the United Kingdom airway responsiveness demonstrated in the laboratory is not often used in the diagnosis of asthma. The clinical equivalent of the increased responsiveness is symptoms that develop in response to dust, smoke, cold air, and exercise; these should be sought in the history.

Labelling

In the past there was a tendency to use the term "wheezy bronchitis" in children rather than "asthma" in the belief that this would protect the parents from the label of asthma. In infants under the age of 2 years wheezing is common because of the small size of the lungs. Many of these affected infants will not go on to wheeze later. In adults who smoke, asthma may be difficult to differentiate from the airway narrowing that is part of chronic bronchitis and emphysema that has been caused by previous cigarette smoking.

The actual diagnostic label would not matter if the appropriate treatment were used. Unfortunately the evidence

The International Consensus Report on the Diagnosis and Management of Asthma[1] gives the following definition. "Asthma is a chronic inflammatory disorder of the airway in which many cells play a role, in particular mast cells, eosinophils, and T lymphocytes. In susceptible individuals this inflammation causes recurrent episodes of wheezing, breathlessness, chest tightness, and cough particularly at night and or in the early morning. These symptoms are usually associated with widespread but variable airflow limitation that is at least partly reversible either spontaneously or with treatment. The inflammation also causes an associated increase in airway responsiveness to a variety of stimuli."

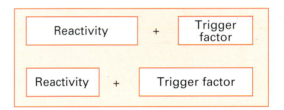

The underlying pathology of asthma is inflammatory change in the airway

THE
PREFACE
TO THE
TREATISE
OF THE
ASTHMA

SINCE the Cure of the *Asthma* is observed by all Physicians, who have attempted the Eradicating that Chronical Distemper, to be very difficult, and frequently unsuccessful; I may thence infer, That either the true Nature of that Disease is not thoroughly understood by them, or they have not yet found out the Medicines by which the Cure may be effected.

It is my Design in this Treatise, to enquire more particularly into the Nature of this Disease; and, according to that Notion I can give of it, to propose those Methods and Medicines which appear to me most likely to effect its Cure, or, at least, to palliate it.

B

The preface to *The Treatise of the Asthma* by J Floyer, published in 1717 shows that children and adults who are diagnosed as having asthma are more likely to get appropriate treatment than children with the same symptoms who are given an alternative label. In adults attempts at bronchodilatation and prophylaxis are more extensive in those who are labelled as asthmatic. Asthma is now such a common and well publicised condition that the diagnosis tends to cause less upset than it used to. With adequate explanation most patients and parents will accept it. The correct treatment can then be started. Persistent problems of cough and wheeze are likely to be much more worrying than the correct diagnosis and improvement in symptoms on treatment. The particular problems of the diagnosis of asthma in very young children are dealt with in chapter 12.

Treating older patients

In older patients with any form of widespread airflow obstruction it is appropriate to try to achieve adequate bronchodilatation, which should be confirmed by objective testing. Prophylaxis with inhaled corticosteroids is well established as an important part of the treatment of asthma. The position of inhaled steroids in chronic obstructive pulmonary disease (COPD) is less certain. There is little evidence of a change in decline of lung function. It is possible that exacerbations might be reduced.

The nature of the airways

The wall of the airway in asthma is thickened by oedema, cellular infiltration, increased smooth muscle, and glands. There is an infiltration by numerous cells, particularly neutrophils and eosinophils, but also lymphocytes and a few mast cells.

Pathology

During the 1990s there has been a far greater emphasis on the inflammatory change than previously. The inflammation in the airway wall involves oedema, infiltration with a variety of cells, disruption and detachment of the epithelial layer, and mucus gland hypertrophy. Changes occur in the subepithelial layer with the laying down of forms of collagen and other extracellular matrix proteins.

This remodelling of the airway wall in response to persistent inflammation can resolve but may result in permanent fibrotic damage thought to be related to the irreversible airflow obstruction that may develop in poorly controlled asthma. Some of the inflammatory changes in the airway wall can be reduced or prevented by suitable therapy. The point when the changes become irreversible is uncertain and an area of considerable interest.

Clinical evidence

Early evidence on the changes in the airway wall came from a few studies of *post mortem* material. The understanding advanced with the use of bronchial biopsies taken at bronchoscopy. These studies showed that, even in remission, there is persistent inflammation in the airway wall. Alveolar lavage produces information on cells in the alveoli and small airways. It is difficult to repeat bronchoscopy often. More recently, sputum induced by breathing hypertonic saline has been used as an alternative.

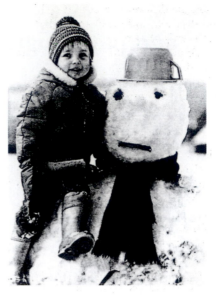

Cold air is a stimulus for asthma Photo: Barnaby's Picture Library

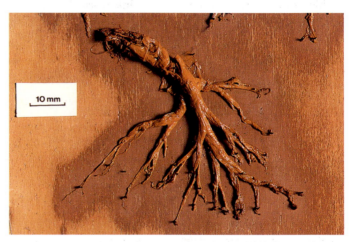

10 mm

Extensive airway plugs and casts of airways can occur in severe asthma

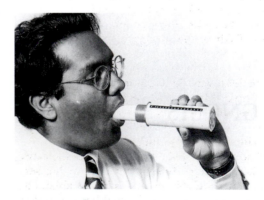

Portable peak flow meters are useful in the diagnosis and monitoring of asthma

Th2 cells, a subgroup of helper T cells, seem to be important co-ordinators of the inflammatory process. The Th2 cells secrete interleukin 4. This stimulates B lymphocytes to generate IgE. Other cytokines such as interleukin 5, interleukin 3 and granulocyte-macrophage colony stimulating factor attract the infiltration of cells such as macrophages, eosinophils and mast cells into the airway wall. These cells in turn release mediators, which are able to continue to augment the inflammatory process

All these techniques sample different areas and cell populations and by themselves may induce changes that affect repeated studies. However, they have provided valuable information on cellular and mediator changes and the effects of treatment or airway challenge. The measurement of exhaled nitric oxide in expired air holds promise for a simpler method of measuring an aspect of airway inflammation.

Mucus plugging

In severe asthma, there is mucus plugging within the lumen and loss of parts of the surface epithelium. Extensive mucus plugging is the striking finding in the lungs of patients who die of an acute exacerbation of asthma.

Asthma as a general condition

It has been suggested that asthma is a generalised abnormality of the inflammatory or immune cells and that the lungs are just the site where the symptoms show. This does not explain the finding that lungs from a donor with mild asthma transplanted into a non-asthmatic produced problems with obstruction of airflow while normal lungs transplanted into an asthmatic patient were free of problems.

Types of asthma

Asthma that develops during childhood usually varies considerably with time and treatment. Most young asthmatic patients have identifiable triggers that provoke wheezing although there is seldom one single extrinsic cause for all their attacks. This "extrinsic" asthma is often associated with other features of atopy such as rhinitis and eczema. When asthma starts in adult life the airflow obstruction is often more persistent and many exacerbations have no obvious stimuli other than respiratory tract infections. This pattern is often called "intrinsic" asthma. Immediate skin prick tests are less likely to be positive because of a lack of involvement of allergens or a loss of skin test positivity with age.

Other categories

There are many patients who do not fit into these broad groups or who overlap the two types. There are other important types of asthma including one that presents with just a cough and one related to occupational exposure.

Presentation with a cough is particularly common in children. Even in adults it should be considered as the cause of chronic unexplained cough. In some series of such cases, asthma, or a combination of rhinitis and asthma, explained the cough in about half the patients who had been troubled by a cough with no obvious cause for more than two months.

References

1. International Consensus Report on the Diagnosis and Management of Asthma. *Clin Exper Allergy* 1992;**22** suppl 1.

Types of asthma

Childhood onset   Usually atopic, tends to have pronounced variability and obvious precipitants
Adult onset   Often more persistent, often few known precipitants except infection
Occupational   Underdiagnosed, needs careful evaluation
Nocturnal   Common in all types, relates to poor overall control and increased reactivity
Cough-variant   May precede airflow obstruction, responds to treatment
Exercise-induced   Common precipitant, may be the main problem in mild cases in children
Brittle   Two types described – chaotic uncontrolled asthma with variable peak flow or severe exacerbations occurring suddenly from a stable baseline

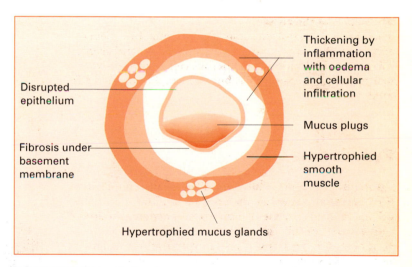

Inflammatory changes in the airway

Differential diagnosis

Chronic bronchitis and emphysema   Difficult to differentiate in older smokers
Large airway obstruction   Caused by foreign bodies and tumours, often misdiagnosed as asthma initially
Pulmonary oedema   So-called "cardiac asthma" – may include wheezing and may also occur at night

2   Prevalence

Genetics

There have been considerable advances in understanding the genetics of asthma over the last few years. A familial link in asthma has been recognised for some time together with an association with allergic rhinitis and allergic eczema. This has been helped by the investigation of isolated communities – such as Tristan da Cunha where the high prevalence of asthma can be traced to three women among the original settlers on the island.

Genetic studies
Early studies of genetic links within families with more than one subject with asthma showed promise of a strong link to certain genetic regions of interest, particularly 5q and 11q. Further studies in different populations did not replicate all the early findings and it became evident that, as in other common conditions, the genetic links were not simple. A number of regions of interest have been detected and there appear to be differences in the links between ethnic groups. Some of the regions of interest are common to the different groups. Some sites are in the region of other possible relevant areas such as the H1A site on chromosome 6 and that controlling IgE production.

The findings fit with a complex disorder with interaction of multiple susceptibility genes. Further studies are needed to look more closely at the regions of interest. The genetic predisposition provided by the combination of interacting genes is then further modulated by environmental influences.

Future investigations
Progress is likely to come from collaborative studies and from further investigation of relatively isolated populations. Members of the Hutterite community in the United States are descendants of 64 individuals who emigrated from Europe in the 17th century. A number of genetic links have been found in this population. Some of the genetic links are related loosely to the atopic phenotype while others appear to link to asthma rather than just atopy.

This remains an exciting field: major advances in therapy still seem some way off but the findings may help in making diagnostic studies, understanding different phenotypes and directing treatments.

Genetic factors and clinical course

Atopic subjects are at risk of asthma and rhinitis; they can be identified by positive immediate skin prick tests to common allergens.

The development of asthma depends on environmental factors acting with a genetic predisposition. The movement of racial groups with a low prevalence of asthma from an isolated rural environment to an urban area increases the prevalence in that group, possibly because of their increased exposure to allergens such as house dust mites and fungal spores or to infectious agents, pollution and dietary changes.

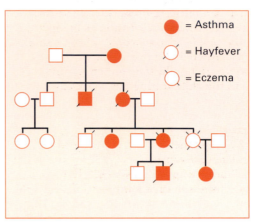

The family tree of an atopic family

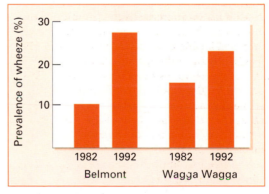

Increase in prevalence of wheeze in 8 to 10 year old children in two towns in New South Wales between 1982 and 1992. There was a pronounced increase in counts of house dust mite in domestic dust over the same period (Peak JK *et al*, *BMJ* 1994;**308**:1591–6)

Family history

The chance of a person developing asthma by the age of 50 years is increased 10 times if there is a first-degree relative with asthma. The risk is greater the more severe the relative's asthma. It has been suggested that breast feeding may reduce the risk of a child developing atopic conditions such as asthma because it restricts the exposure to ingested foreign protein in the first few months of life. Conflicting studies have been published and it may require considerable dietary restriction by the mother to avoid passing antigen on to the child during this vulnerable period.

Smoking in pregnancy

Maternal smoking in pregnancy increases the risk of childhood asthma; exposure during the first few years of life is also detrimental. Studies of paternal smoking have produced less certain trends in the same direction.

Weight control

A number of studies have shown that obesity is associated with an increased likelihood of asthma. Regular exercise to maintain fitness and control weight is sensible advice for asthmatics.

Prevalence figures

The reported prevalence depends on the definition of asthma being used and the age and type of the population being studied. Although changes in criteria and fashions make interpretation difficult a number of studies have suggested that there is a slow increase in the prevalence of asthma in most countries. There are regional variations, particularly among developing countries where the rates in urban areas are higher than in the poor rural districts. In developed countries there is no association with social class except a tendency to give the label of asthma more readily to those in social classes I and II.

Most studies that have used equivalent diagnostic criteria in a stable group have suggested that the prevalence is increasing. This is more difficult to judge in young children and in subjects over 50 years old when differential diagnoses produce uncertainty. The results fit in with other information such as the data on hospital admissions and general practitioners' workload with asthmatic patients. In the United States asthma is more prevalent among blacks than whites but in the United Kingdom the association is less pronounced.

In children the prevalence of asthma in the 5 to 12 year age group is over 10%. Australian studies give a prevalence nearer 20%. The sex ratio in children aged around 7 years shows that one and a half times to twice as many boys are affected as girls, but during their teenage years boys do better than girls and by the time they reach adulthood the sex incidence has become about equal.

Incidence of wheezing

Wheezing is a common symptom; questionnaires have shown that about 30% of the population wheezes at some time. In many cases the wheezing is temporary and develops in otherwise normal subjects after a viral infection. The inflammation of the airway leaves nerve endings exposed and vulnerable to the effects of potentially harmful stimuli such as smoke and dust particles.

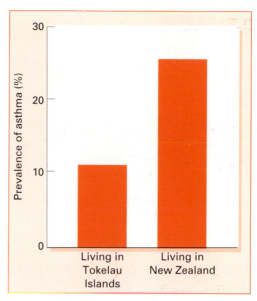

Prevalence of asthma in Tokelauan children aged 0 to 14 years still in the Tokelau Islands or resettled in New Zealand. Asthma, rhinitis, and eczema were all more prevalent in islanders who had been resettled in New Zealand after a hurricane. Environmental factors have an effect as well as genetic predisposition (Waite DA *et al*, *Clinical Allergy* 1980;**10**:71–5)

Diagnostic criteria in epidemiological studies

For epidemiological purposes, a common set of criteria is the presence of symptoms during the previous 12 months, together with evidence of increased bronchial responsiveness. More reliable information about asthma and allergy symptoms in children from more than 50 countries will come from the International Study of Asthma and Allergies in Childhood (ISAAC).

The Odense study in children[1] found 27% with current asthma symptoms but only 10% diagnosed as asthmatic. Different diagnostic tests such as methacholine responsiveness, peak flow monitoring and exercise testing did not correlate well with each other. Each test was reasonably specific but individual sensitivities tended to be low. In this study the combination of peak flow monitoring at home and methacholine responsiveness produced the best results. The results confirm that no single physiological test is perfect and suggest that the different tests may detect different clinical aspects of asthma. A positive result in either test with a typical history would confirm the diagnosis of asthma.

Increase in prevalence

A number of explanations have been put forward for the increase in the prevalence of asthma. The strong genetic element has not changed so any true increase outside changes in detection or diagnosis must come from environmental factors. No single explanation is likely to provide the complete answer since the likely factors do not apply equally to all the populations experiencing the change in prevalence. Explanations for the increase in the prevalence of asthma include:

Change in the indoor environment
The advent of centrally heated homes with warm bedrooms full of soft furnishings is likely to increase the exposure to house dust mite. Exposure of the immature immune system of infants to these allergens may set up sensitivities that manifest later as asthma.

Smoking
Maternal smoking during pregnancy and infancy is associated with an increased prevalence of asthma in childhood. The increase in smoking among young women in recent years may play some part in the increase in prevalence.

Infections
Epidemiological studies show a higher prevalence of asthma in first-born children. This is thought to be related to a higher exposure to common viruses in infancy when siblings are present. Such infections may help to mature the immune system changing undifferentiated lymphocytes to the Th1 rather than Th2 type associated with IgE production. Thus a general reduction in family sizes will increase the prevalence of asthma.

Diet
A number of studies have shown relationships between diet and asthma related to higher salt intake, low selenium or reduced vitamin C.

Reference
1. Siersted HC, Mostgaard G, Hyldebrandt N, Hansen HS, Boldsen J, Oxhoj H. Interrelationships between diagnosed asthma, asthma-like symptoms, and abnormal airway behaviour in adolescence: the Odense Schoolchild Study. *Thorax* 1996;**51**:503–9.

3 Diagnostic testing and monitoring

Recording airflow obstruction

Mini peak flow meters provide a cheap method of measuring airflow obstruction. Several types are available on prescription. They may have errors that vary over the range of measurement but patients using the same peak flow meter over time can build up a pattern of their asthma, which can be important in changing their treatment and planning management. The measurements add an objective element to subjective feelings of shortness of breath.

Use of diary cards

Although acute attacks of asthma occasionally have a sudden catastrophic onset they are more usually preceded by a gradual deterioration in control, which may not be noticed until it is quite advanced. An appreciable minority of patients, probably 15 to 20%, will be unaware of moderate changes in their airflow obstruction even when these occur acutely; these patients are at particular risk of an acute exacerbation without warning. When such patients are identified they should be encouraged to take regular peak flow recordings and enter them on a diary card, to permit them to see trends in peak flow measurements and react to exacerbations at an early stage before there is any change in their symptoms.

Treatment plans

Mini peak flow meters are inexpensive and have an important role in educating patients about their asthma. They should be used much more widely than they are and should be regarded as the equivalent in asthma of the regular urine or blood testing common among diabetic patients. It is not enough simply to give out a peak flow meter. Based on the home recordings, the doctor and the asthmatic patient can work together to develop plans with criteria that indicate the need for a change in treatment, a visit to the doctor, or emergency admission to hospital. This management plan should be written down for the patient and should be reviewed periodically.

It has not been possible to show an effect on the control of asthma or hospital admission from the use of a peak flow meter alone, but a personal asthma management plan supported by regular follow up does improve control. This may involve twice daily peak flow recordings but many asthmatics find it difficult to perform this in practice.

Responsiveness to bronchodilators

Responses to bronchodilators are easy to measure in the clinic or surgery. Reversibility is often used to establish the diagnosis of asthma or to find out which is the most effective bronchodilator. Because of the variability in asthma, airflow obstruction may not be present at the time of testing. Reversibility is relatively specific but not very sensitive as a diagnostic test in mild asthma.

Measuring reversibility

Reversibility is usually assessed by recording the best of three peak flow measurements and repeating the measurements 15 to 30 minutes after the patient has

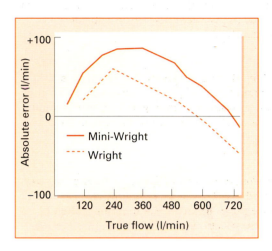

Errors in readings of Mini-Wright and Wright peak flow meters compared with flow from a pneumotachograph. Both over-read at lower flow rates and are non-linear (Miller RD *et al*, *Thorax* 1992;**47**:904–9)

Particular encouragement to record peak flow should be given to:
- Poor perceivers, where symptoms do not reflect changes in objective measured obstruction
- Patients with a history of sudden exacerbations
- Patients with poor asthma control
- Times of adjustment in therapy either up or down
- Situations where a precipitating event is suspected
- Periodic recordings in stable asthma to establish usual levels and confirm reliability of symptoms

---

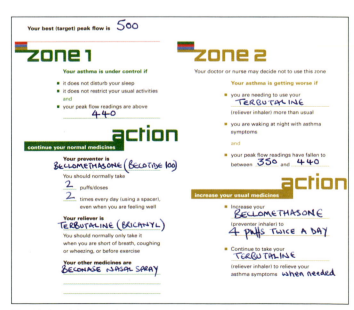

The National Asthma Campaign produces a self management plan in the form of a leaflet that can be completed for each patient

inhaled two or more doses of a β-agonist, salbutamol or terbutaline from a metered dose inhaler or dry powder system. The method of inhalation should be supervised and the opportunity taken to correct the technique or change to a different inhalation device if necessary. The 95% confidence intervals for a change in peak flow rate on such repetitions are around 60 to 70 l/min.

When forced expiratory volume in one second (FEV_1) is the measurement used, a change of 200 ml is outside the variability of the test. A standard dose of a β-agonist can be combined with an anticholinergic agent – ipratropium or oxitropium bromide. These agents are slower to act than β-agonists and their effect should be assessed 40 to 60 minutes after inhalation.

When there is severe obstruction and reversibility is limited, application of strict reversibility criteria may be inappropriate for the purpose of determining treatments. Any response may be worthwhile so attention should be paid to subjective responses and improvement of exercise tolerance together with results of other tests of respiratory function. Reversibility shown by other tests such as those of lung volumes or trapped gas volumes without changes in peak flow or FEV_1 are more likely to occur in patients with COPD than in those with asthma.

Further review

Decisions about treatment from such single dose studies should be backed up by further objective and subjective measurements during long-term treatment. Responses to bronchodilators are not always consistent and, in some patients, changes after single doses in the laboratory may not predict the responses to the same drug over more prolonged periods.

Peak flow variation

A characteristic of asthma is a cyclical variation in the degree of airflow obstruction throughout the day. The lowest peak flow values occur in the early hours of the morning and the highest occur in the afternoon. To see the pattern a peak flow meter should be used at least twice and up to four times a day. A difference of at least 15% between mean morning and evening values is diagnostic of asthma. Many reasons have been suggested involving diurnal variation in adrenaline, vagal activity, cortisol, airway inflammation and β_2-receptor function changes.

Diurnal variation

Documentation of diurnal variation by recording measurements from a peak flow meter shows typical diagnostic patterns in many patients. The timing of the measurements should be recorded, otherwise typical variations can be obscured by later readings at the weekend or on days away from work or school.

In non-asthmatic subjects there is a small degree of diurnal variation with the same timing. A strict definition of diurnal variation does not correlate very well with other diagnostic tests in asthma. A looser definition – minimum peak flow of less than 80% maximum over two weeks of recordings – may be more reliable.

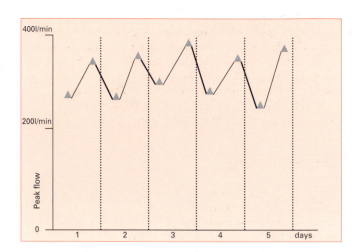

Diurnal percentage variation in peak flow readings
Mean daily variation [(maximum−minimum)÷maximum]=24%

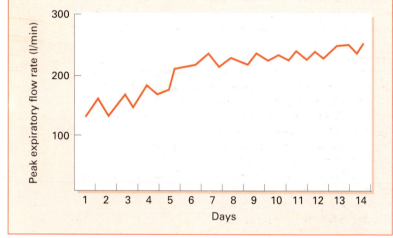

Peak flow during a two week course of oral corticosteroids in persistent asthma. The response levels out on days 9 and 10

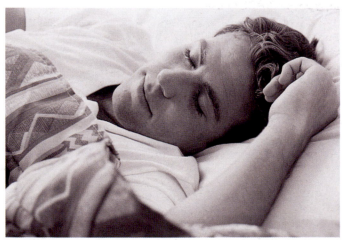

The lowest peak flow values occur in the early hours of the morning
Photo: The Stock Market

Nocturnal attacks

People with asthma commonly complain of waking at night. Large studies in the United Kingdom suggest that more than half of those with asthma have their sleep disturbed by an attack more than once a week. Questions about sleep disturbance by breathlessness and cough should be asked routinely in consultations with asthmatic patients. Deaths from asthma are also more likely to occur in the early hours of the morning.

Exercise testing

The provocation test most often used in the United Kingdom is a simple exercise test.

Exercise testing is a safe, simple procedure and may be useful when the diagnosis of asthma is in doubt. Non-asthmatic patients do not develop bronchoconstriction on exercise; indeed, they usually show a small degree of bronchodilatation during the exercise itself. When baseline lung function is low, provocation testing is unnecessary for diagnosis as reversibility can be shown by bronchodilatation.

Exercise testing and the recording of diurnal variations are used when the history suggests asthma but lung function is normal when the patient is seen. An exercise test may consist of baseline peak flow measurements, then six minutes of vigorous exercise such as running, followed by peak flow measurements for 20 minutes afterwards.

Testing outdoors

The exercise is best done outside because breathing cold, dry air intensifies the response. The characteristic asthmatic response is a fall in peak flow of more than 15% several minutes after the end of exercise. About 90% of asthmatic children will show a drop in peak flow in response to exercise. Once the peak flow rate has fallen by 15% the bronchoconstriction should be reversed by inhalation of a bronchodilator. Late reactions about six hours after challenge are unusual; unlike challenge with an allergen, patients do not need to be kept under observation for late responses after the initial response has been reversed. Such exercise tests are best avoided if the patient has ischaemic heart disease, but there is no reason why peak flow measurements should not be included during supervised exercise testing for coronary artery disease where this is appropriate.

Other types of challenge

The exercise test relies on changes in temperature and in the osmolality of the airway mucosa. Other challenge tests that rely on similar mechanisms include isocapnic hyperventilation; breathing cold, dry air; and osmotic challenge with nebulised distilled water or hypertonic saline. These are, however, laboratory-based procedures whereas the simple exercise test for asthma can be done at any clinic or surgery.

Bronchodilators and sodium cromoglycate should be stopped at least six hours before the exercise test and long acting oral or inhaled bronchodilators should be stopped for at least 24 hours.

Leukotriene antagonists are effective in blocking exercise-induced asthma but are unlikely to be relevant to a diagnostic exercise test. Similarly, prolonged use of inhaled corticosteroids reduces responses to exercise but these are not usually stopped before testing because the effect takes days or weeks to wear off.

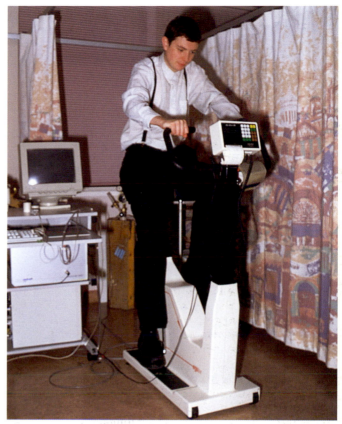

Exercise test on a treadmill

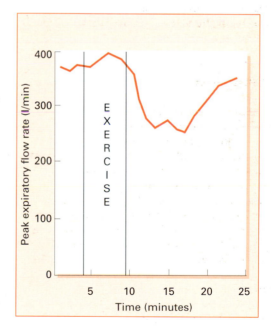

Decrease in peak expiratory flow rate in response to exercise

Airway hyperresponsiveness

Other common forms of non-specific challenge to the airways are the inhalation of methacholine and histamine. These tests produce a range of responses usually defined as the dose of the challenging agent necessary to produce a drop in the FEV_1 of 20%. This is calculated by giving increasing doses until the FEV_1 drops below 80% of the baseline measurement, then drawing a line to connect the last two points above and below a 20% drop and taking the dose at the point on this line equivalent to a 20% drop in FEV_1. Nearly all patients with asthma show increased responsiveness, whereas patients with hayfever and not asthma form an intermediate group.

This responsiveness of asthmatic patients has been associated with the underlying inflammation in the airway wall. Such non-specific bronchial challenge is performed as an outpatient procedure in hospital respiratory function units. It is a safe procedure providing it is monitored carefully and not used in the presence of moderately severe airflow obstruction.

Degree of responsiveness

The degree of responsiveness is associated with the severity of the airways disease. It can be reduced by strict avoidance of known allergens. Drugs such as corticosteroids reduce responsiveness through their effect on inflammation in the wall of the airway but they do not usually return reactivity to the normal range. Use of a bronchodilator is followed by a temporary reduction while the mechanisms of smooth muscle contraction are blocked. Bronchial reactivity is an important epidemiological and research tool. In clinical practice its use varies widely between countries. It is most useful where there are difficult diagnostic problems such as persistent cough.

Specific airway challenge

Challenge with specific agents to which a patient is thought to be sensitive must be done with caution. The initial dose should be low and, even so, reactions may be unpredictable. Early narrowing of the airway by contraction of smooth muscle occurs within the first 30 minutes and there is often a "late response" four to eight hours later.

The late response may be followed by poorer control of the asthma and greater diurnal variation for days or weeks afterwards. The late response is thought to be associated with release of mediators and attraction of inflammatory cells to the airways. It has been used in drug development as a more suitable model for clinical asthma than the brief early response.

Challenges with specific allergens are used mostly for the investigation of occupational asthma but they should be restricted to experienced laboratories. Patients should be supervised for at least eight hours after challenge.

Skin tests

In skin prick tests a small amount of the test substance is introduced into the superficial layers of the epidermis on the tip of a small needle. The tests are painless, just causing

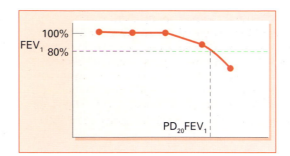

Log dose of histamine or methacholine

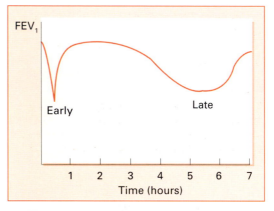

Drop in FEV_1 in a bronchial reactivity test

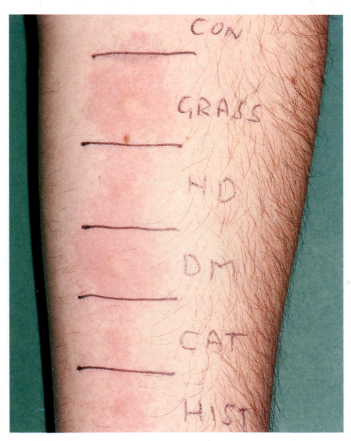

Skin prick tests. This patient is being exposed to a range of common allergens

temporary local itching. More general reactions are theoretically possible but extremely rare. Most young asthmatics show a range of positive responses to common allergens such as house dust mite, pollens and animal dander. A weal that develops 15 minutes after a skin prick test suggests the presence of specific IgE antibody; the results correlate well with those of *in vitro* tests for IgE such as the radioallergosorbent test, which is more expensive.

Atopy

Positive skin tests do not establish a diagnosis of asthma or the importance of the specific allergens used. They show only the tendency to produce IgE to common allergens – confirming atopy. More than 20% of the population have positive skin tests, but less than a half of these will develop asthma. The prevalence and strength of positive skin tests declines with age. The pattern of skin test responses depends on prior exposure and, therefore, varies with geography and social factors.

Importance of history

The importance of allergic factors in asthma is best ascertained from a careful clinical history, taking into account seasonal factors and trials of avoidance of allergens. Suspicions can be confirmed by skin tests or, less often, by specific inhalation challenge.

Conclusions

Although positive skin tests do not incriminate the allergen as a cause of the patient's asthma it would be rare for an inhalant to be important in asthma with a negative skin test. The results do, however, rely on the quality of the agents used in testing and will be negative if antihistamines are being taken. Corticosteroids have no appreciable effect on immediate skin prick tests.

Differential diagnosis

The difficulty in breathing that is characteristic of asthma may be described as a constriction in the chest that suggests ischaemic cardiac pain. Nocturnal asthma that causes the patient to be woken from sleep by breathlessness may be confused with the paroxysmal nocturnal dyspnoea of heart failure.

Asthma and COPD

After some years, particularly when it is severe, asthma may lose some or all of its reversibility. COPD, usually caused by cigarette smoking, may show appreciable reversibility, which can make it quite difficult to be sure of the correct diagnosis in older patients with partially reversible obstruction. Evidence is emerging that the pathological changes in the airway may be different in asthma and COPD.

However, in practice, bronchodilators are given and corticosteroids used to establish the best airway function that can be achieved. Some studies suggested that inhaled steroids slow the rate of decline of lung function with age in COPD but this has not been confirmed in larger studies in mild to moderate COPD. There may be a reduction in exacerbations but more work is needed before they can be regarded as part of the routine treatment of COPD. Meanwhile when there is reversibility to bronchodilators and any doubt whether the diagnosis might be asthma, then inhaled corticosteroids should be part of the treatment.

Non-asthmatic wheezing

Other causes of wheezing, such as obstruction of the large airways, occasionally produce problems in diagnosis. This may be the case with foreign bodies, particularly in children, or with tumours that gradually obstruct the trachea or main airways in adults. The noise produced is often a single pitched wheeze on inspiration and expiration rather than the multiple expiratory wheezes typical of asthma. Appropriate X-rays and flow volume loops can show the site of obstruction. On spirometry the volume time curve may be a straight line.

Vocal cord dysfunction

Some patients have upper airway obstruction at laryngeal level produced apparently by dysfunction of the vocal cord musculature. The obstruction is most evident in inspiration and may show as premature termination of inspiration in the flow volume loop. The phenomenon seems to be more common in young women; it is often mistaken for or coincident with asthma and can be difficult to treat.

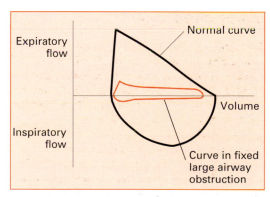

Flow–volume curve

4 Clinical course

"Growing out" of asthma

Parents of asthmatic children are usually concerned about whether their child will "grow out of" asthma. Most wheezy children improve during their teens but the outlook depends to some extent on the severity of their early disease.

Over half the children whose wheezing is infrequent will be free of symptoms by the time they are 21 years old, but of those with frequent, troublesome wheezing only 20% will be symptom free at 21, although 20% will be substantially better. In 15% of patients, asthma becomes more troublesome in early adult years than it was in childhood. Even if there is prolonged remission lasting several years symptoms may return later. After months free of symptoms, biopsy studies show that the airway epithelium may still be inflamed and airway responsiveness to methacholine and histamine may remain abnormally high. This suggests that the underlying tendency to be asthmatic remains and a third of the children who have a year's remission will get further symptoms years later.

Likelihood of remission

Asthma is less likely to go into remission in patients with a strong family history of atopy or a personal history of other atopic conditions, low respiratory function, onset after the age of 29 and frequent attacks. More boys than girls are affected by asthma but the girls do less well during adolescence and by adulthood the sex ratio is equal. Most of those who do grow out of asthma are left with no residual effects other than the risk of recrudescence. Chest deformities are uncommon and only occur when there is severe, intractable disease.

Adult height

Although puberty may be delayed, the final adult height of children with asthma is usually normal unless they have received long-term treatment with systemic or high-dose inhaled corticosteroids.

Prognosis in adults

Asthma in adults often shows less spontaneous variation than it does in children. Wheezing is more persistent and there is less association with obvious precipitating factors other than infections. The chances of a sustained remission are also lower than in children. Smokers with increased bronchial reactivity are particularly at risk of developing chronic airflow obstruction and it is vital that asthmatic patients do not smoke. When there are known precipitating agents that can be avoided – such as animals or occupational factors – then sustained removal of these will reduce bronchial reactivity. The avoidance of contact with known allergens can decrease the inflammation in the airway wall and thus reduce responses to non-specific agents including cigarette smoke, cold air, and dust. It can lead to an improvement in the control and the progress of the asthma.

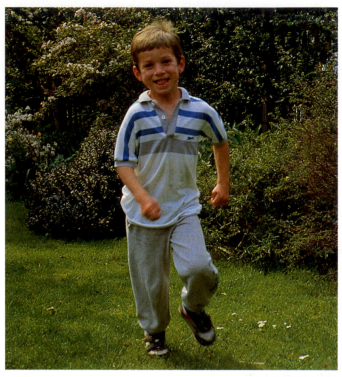

Parents hope that their children's asthma will improve as they get older

---

Asthma: things to avoid

- Known allergens
- Active and passive cigarette smoking
- Areas of high pollution (particularly exercise at times of high air pollution)
- β-blockers
- Aspirin and non-steroidal anti-inflammatory drugs
- Obesity

The reversibility of airway obstruction in asthma is not always maintained throughout life. Those with more severe asthma are most likely to go on to develop irreversible airflow obstruction. It is likely that this progression to irreversibility is related to persistent inflammation of the wall of the airway, which leads to permanent damage. Suitable prolonged prophylaxis reduces the inflammation and most chest physicians act on the belief that this will reduce the likelihood of long-term damage and eventual irreversibility. There are few prolonged studies to prove or disprove this contention but the benefits of anti-inflammatory prophylaxis are well established in the short term and it seems prudent to follow this practice.

A few studies around introduction of inhaled corticosteroids give some hope that treatment can affect the clinical course. The degree of impairment in lung function on starting inhaled steroids is greatest in those with the shortest history of symptoms, suggesting that more prolonged untreated disease may lead to irreversible change. Delayed onset of inhaled steroids in one study comparing β-agonists and steroids seemed to reduce the potential benefit of the steroids. Set against these studies are the changes seen at the end of trials of inhaled steroids. Bronchial responsiveness and lung function seem to return to baseline rapidly.

This is an important area for further study with implications for the stage to start inhaled steroids; the relative position in treatment of bronchodilators, steroids and other agents such as cromoglycate, theophylline and leukotriene antagonists and the approach to treatment once control is achieved.

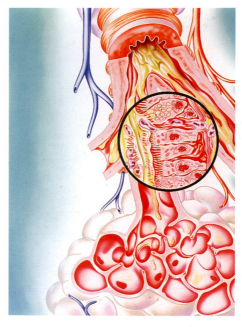

Cut away illustration of the respiratory system showing changes in severe asthma. A trigger such as an infection or allergen causes widespread airway narrowing through inflammation and bronchoconstriction. In addition goblet cells produce excess sticky mucus which can obstruct airways. Such mucus plugging is a prominent feature in fatal cases of asthma Credit: Science Photo Library

Deaths from asthma

Since the sharp temporary increase in mortality from asthma seen in some countries during the early 1960s there has been concern about the role of treatment in such deaths. The deaths in the 1960s have been attributed to cardiac stimulation caused by overuse of inhaled isoprenaline, or to excessive reliance on its usual efficacy leading to delay in using appropriate alternative treatment when symptoms worsened. Isoprenaline as a bronchodilator has been superseded by safer β_2-stimulants.

Mortality in the United Kingdom
After the peak in the 1960s, the number of deaths from asthma in the United Kingdom stabilised. In the late 1980s there was a suggestion of a gradual rise in deaths to about 2000 per year but statistics for the 1990s show a gradual decline in mortality. The figures are most reliable for the 5 to 34 year age range and the most recent figures confirm a slight fall in mortality in the group.

Mortality in New Zealand
In the 1980s mortality from asthma in New Zealand rose appreciably. Once again the reasons are uncertain and have aroused controversy. The increase in deaths in New Zealand has been reversed and has not been mirrored elsewhere. The combination of methylxanthines and β_2-stimulants – and the use of home nebulisers – were blamed but neither provided a satisfactory explanation for the problems. In New Zealand fenoterol was a popular β_2-agonist and it has

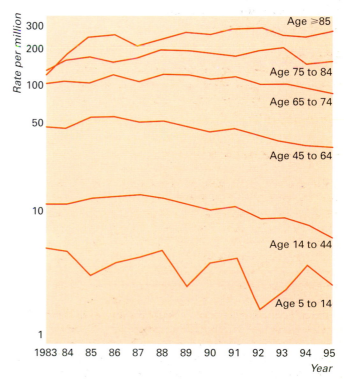

Death rates from asthma per million population by age group, from a study in England and Wales[1]

been linked to the increase in mortality because it is claimed that it has more cardiac stimulating effects than other β_2-agonists and that it was marketed in a higher strength dose for dose than in the United Kingdom.

An alternative suggestion was that it was used in more severe cases, but an attempt to explore this hypothesis by retrospective case matching did not support the explanation. These doubts fuelled worries about the possibility that β_2-agonists might have the potential to worsen control of asthma and increase morbidity and even mortality. Further studies on regular short acting β-agonists and trials of up to 12 months of long acting β-agonists have failed to confirm the problems of regular usage.

Need for rapid response

Investigation of the circumstances surrounding individual deaths generally finds evidence of under-treatment rather than excessive medication in such deaths. Doctors and patients underestimate the severity of attacks; the most important factor may be an apparent reluctance to take oral corticosteroids for severe asthmatic episodes and to adjust treatment early during periods of deterioration. Nevertheless, about a quarter of deaths occur less than an hour after the start of an exacerbation. Patients who have such rapid deterioration are particularly vulnerable. If patients have deteriorated swiftly in the past they should have suitable treatment readily available, such as steroids and nebulised and injectable bronchodilators. Patients and their relatives must be confident in the use of their emergency treatment and know how to obtain further help immediately.

Several centres have adopted the policy of maintaining a self admission service for selected asthmatic patients. This avoids delay in admitting patients to hospital and is a logical development of involving patients in the management of their own disease.

Diurnal variation

Some studies have shown that patients are particularly at risk after they have been discharged from intensive care or high dependency units to ordinary wards, and after discharge from hospital. Problems often occur in the early hours of the morning at the nadir of the diurnal cycle. They may be related to premature tailing off of the initial intensive treatment because the measurements during the day have been satisfactory. Monitoring of peak flow will identify the instability of the asthma manifested by a large diurnal variability in peak flow. Adequate supervision and treatment must be maintained throughout these periods until control is restored.

British Thoracic Society guidelines

Assessment and management in hospital have also been criticised. Asthma has proved to be a popular subject for audit according to the consensus guidelines of the British Thoracic Society (BTS). Many studies have shown that initial assessment and treatment are satisfactory but that there are weaknesses in the exploration of reasons for an attack, establishment of adequate control before discharge, and follow up arrangements. Every admission should be regarded as a failure of routine management. The usual treatment, compliance with therapy and the existence and performance of management plans should be explored with

> **The most important element in asthma fatalities is lack of appreciation of severity by the patient or doctor, leading to under-treatment**

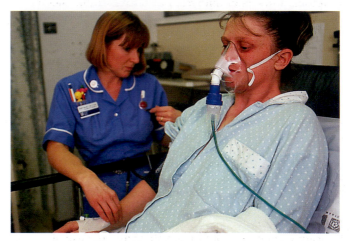

Asthma patient in emergency department

Categories of drug used in asthma

For relief
  Inhaled β-agonists
  Inhaled anticholinergics
  Regular bronchodilators
  Theophyllines
  Oral β-agonists
  Long acting β-agonists
For prophylaxis
  Inhaled corticosteroids
  Sodium cromoglycate
  Nedocromil sodium
  Leukotriene receptor antagonists

the patient. Quality of treatment, readmission rates and asthma control are improved when the inpatient care is supervised by those with an interest in thoracic medicine. Admission to hospital may be an appropriate opportunity to involve a respiratory nurse specialist in the management.

Morbidity

Asthma causes considerable morbidity with persistent symptoms and loss of time from work and school. Sleep is disturbed by asthma more than once a week in over 50% of patients and this leads to poorer daytime performance. There has been a shift in the general approach to management aiming to produce freedom from symptoms, rather than a tolerable existence free of disabling attacks. The aims of the first three steps of the British Thoracic Society guidelines involve virtual freedom from symptoms with minimal or no use of rescue bronchodilator. In children this would include freedom to take part in regular exercise. This requires a more aggressive approach early in the course of the disease with regular anti-inflammatory drugs and will, it is hoped, lead to a reduction in morbidity from exacerbations of asthma and long-term damage.

Patient education
Educating patients about their asthma and the use of treatment is an integral part of management. Patients forget much of what they are told in consultations and information should be backed up by written instructions. It is often helpful to produce these individually for each patient. Standard written information from asthma societies and other sources can be used as a backup, but a personal plan is preferable and can be produced from simple word processor templates. Patients are often confused about the differences between regular prophylaxis, such as inhaled corticosteroids or sodium cromoglycate, and the quickly effective inhaled bronchodilators used to treat acute attacks.

Regular use of a mini peak flow meter allows the patient to participate more effectively in the understanding and treatment of the disease. Even with this information, though, many patients do not adhere to their prescribed regimen. Only half of all asthmatic patients achieve 75% compliance with their prescribed treatment. This is true for all chronic conditions and shows the need for regular reinforcement (matching the information to the patients) and for further work in the area of education and compliance. Development of these management plans requires time, reinforcing and extending the information on repeat visits.

Reference
1. Campbell MJ, Cogman GR, Holgate ST, Johnston SL. Age specific trends in asthma mortality in England and Wales, 1983–95: results of an observational study. *BMJ* 1997;**314**:1439–41.

Individual management plan

Prevention
- Take the budesonide once in the morning and once at night every day
- If you get a cold or peak flow drops below 300 l/min take two doses morning and night

Relief
- Take the salbutamol (two puffs) when you need it
- If you need it more than five times a day get an appointment

Action
- Peak flow less than 250 l/min – start prednisolone six tablets a day and get an appointment within 48 hours
- Peak flow less than 200 l/min and wheezy – take six prednisolone tablets, four puffs of salbutamol, and ring the surgery or go to casualty

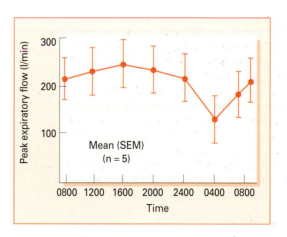

Peak flow measurements can be used to confirm the diagnosis of nocturnal asthma. Decreases in the early hours are associated with disturbed sleep and daytime tiredness (Shapiro C, ed, *ABC of Sleep Disorders*, BMJ Books, London, 1993:52)

5 Precipitating factors

Bronchial hyperresponsiveness

The concept of increased reactivity of the airway to specific and non-specific stimuli is discussed in chapter 2. While inflammatory change in the airway wall is associated with increased reactivity, the underlying mechanisms of increased bronchial reactivity are uncertain. The sustained reactivity found in asthmatic patients has been attributed to imbalance of autonomic control or other non-adrenergic, non-cholinergic plexuses, abnormal immunological and cellular responses, increased permeability of the epithelium and intrinsic differences in the action of smooth muscle or its hypertrophy.

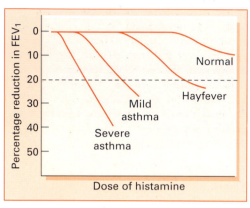

Bronchial reactivity is increased in asthma, particularly in more severe disease

Non-specific stimuli
Airways in asthmatic patients are usually sensitive to non-specific stimuli such as dust and smoke. Laughing or coughing may provoke wheezing. Specific responses to agents such as pollen may lead to increased non-specific reactivity and symptoms of asthma for days or even weeks. Upper respiratory viral infections may lead to similar changes and may increase reactivity in non-asthmatic subjects. In contrast, avoidance of exposure to known allergens may lead to improved control of asthma with reduced responses to other stimuli. Challenge to airways by specific allergens may induce late responses six to ten hours after exposure. Such late responses may mimic more closely the inflammatory changes caused by asthma that occur spontaneously. They lead to a subsequent rise in non-specific airway reactivity.

Exercise

Vigorous exercise produces narrowing of the airways in most asthmatic patients and – as described in chapter 2 – can be used as a simple diagnostic test. Asthma during or after exercise is most likely to be a practical problem in children, where it may interfere with games at school. The type of exercise influences the response; most asthmatic patients find that swimming in warm indoor pools is the activity least likely to induce an attack. This observation has been explained by clinical studies showing the importance of cooling and drying of the airways during hyperventilation and exercise. The effect of exercise can be mimicked by breathing cold, dry air, whereas breathing warm, humid air – as in indoor swimming pools – prevents the asthmatic response. In some patients, however, this picture is confused, because they are sensitive to the chemical agents used in swimming pools.

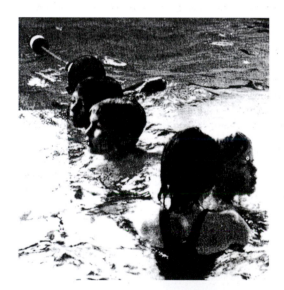

Pre-medication with a β_2-stimulant or sodium cromoglycate usually allows asthmatic children to participate in sports

Drug prophylaxis
Protection against exercise-induced asthma is provided by many of the commonly used drugs. Use of a short acting β_2-agonist 15 to 30 minutes before exercise is usually effective. Sodium cromoglycate and nedocromil sodium also block the response and such treatments will normally allow a child to take part in games at school. Long acting

β$_2$-agonists and leukotriene receptor antagonists are effective in preventing or minimising exercise induced asthma. It may be necessary to explain to teachers the use of drugs and the objectives of the treatment.

Exercise itself is unlikely to have any major beneficial effect on asthma, but general fitness and weight control should be encouraged. A fit person can do a given task with less overall ventilation than an unfit one – hence the reduced likelihood of exercise-induced asthma. Asthma is quite compatible with a successful sporting career, as a number of athletes have testified, and the common inhaled asthma drugs are allowed in the regulations of most sporting bodies. The exceptions are fenoterol and a compound that includes isoprenaline.

Refractoriness

A second bout of exercise within an hour or so of the first is often less troublesome, a phenomenon known as refractoriness. The general benefits of warming up before exercise may therefore be increased for asthmatic athletes. Late asthmatic responses four to six hours after exposure are common after exposure to allergens, but they are rare and not troublesome after exercise.

Allergens in the home

The house dust mite, *Dermatophagoides pteronyssinus*, provides the material for the most common positive skin prick test in the United Kingdom. The main allergen is found in the mites' faecal pellets. The mites live off human skin scales; are widely distributed in bedding, furniture, carpets and soft toys; and thrive best in warm, damp conditions. The expectation of a warm environment at home has increased the exposure of children to allergens and is likely to be an important element in the increased prevalence of asthma.

Change of environment

If patients move into environments that are free of house dust mites their symptoms improve. This can be achieved in the mountains of Switzerland or, near to home but less picturesque, in specially cleaned hospital wards without soft furnishings.

It is more difficult to reduce the numbers of mites sufficiently in the home. Regular cleaning of bedrooms and avoiding materials that are particularly likely to collect dust are sensible measures to keep down the antigenic load.

Substantial reduction in mite antigen is possible by reducing the amount of soft furnishing, extensive cleaning, and the use of mattress covers made of materials such as Gortex, which are impermeable to mites. Acaricides, or even applications of liquid nitrogen to mattresses, can produce a temporary drop. Vacuum cleaners fitted with fine filters may help, in combination with measures that address reservoirs of antigen in sites such as mattresses. Although these measures reduce mite numbers they have not been shown to be effective in asthma control, probably because they do not produce enough of a sustained reduction in house dust mite antigen. Desensitisation to house dust mites may be of some use in children.

Cockroaches

Recent studies have shown high levels of sensitivity to cockroach allergen in some areas. These levels are around 50% in institutions and lower socio-economic groups.

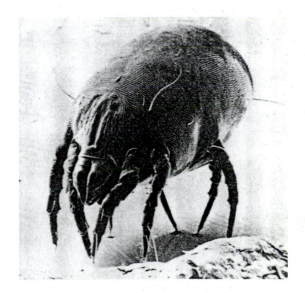

Electron micrograph of a house dust mite

17

Pollens and spores

Seasonal asthma, often together with rhinitis and conjunctivitis, is most usually associated with grass pollens, which are most common during June and July. Less common in the United Kingdom is precipitation of asthma by tree pollens, many of which are produced between February and May, and mould spores from *Cladosporium* and *Alternaria*, which abound in July and August. Complete avoidance of such widespread pollens is impractical.

Hyposensitisation
The effectiveness of hyposensitisation is debatable. It is generally unnecessary because inhaled drugs usually produce adequate control and are simple to use. The strong placebo effect, allergic reactions to hyposensitisation and the occasional mortality must also be taken into account in assessing its value.

Allergic bronchopulmonary aspergillosis

Some asthmatic patients develop a sensitivity to the spores of *Aspergillus fumigatus*, which is a common fungus particularly partial to rotting vegetation. Allergic bronchopulmonary aspergillosis is associated with eosinophilia in blood and sputum, rubbery brownish plugs of mucus containing fungal hyphae and proximal bronchiectasis. Areas of consolidation and collapse may be visible in the chest X-ray film and each episode can lead to further bronchiectatic damage. The Aspergillus skin test will be positive and specific IgE will be found in the blood.

Individual episodes settle after treatment with corticosteroids but if they are frequent and bronchiectasis is developing then long-term oral corticosteroids may be appropriate. Antifungal imidazoles such as itraconazole may also reduce the frequency of attacks.

Pets

The parents of asthmatic children often worry about household pets. Cats cause the greatest problem, with allergens in saliva, urine and dander, but most domestic animals can trigger asthma on occasions. Associated symptoms of conjunctivitis and rhinitis are very common. Patients who have major problems with their asthma should be advised not to acquire any new pets.

When children are born into a family with a strong history of atopy, furry and hairy pets are best avoided. Pets already in residence should be kept out of bedrooms and off soft furnishings. If the animal seems to be a cause of serious symptoms, a trial separation should be organised. Animal allergens remain in the house long after the pet is removed so the pet should move out for a month or two; alternatively the patient could move out for a week or two. Unjustified removal of favourite pets without good reason may, however, provoke more serious problems from emotional upset.

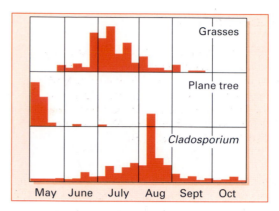

Seasonal variations in allergens

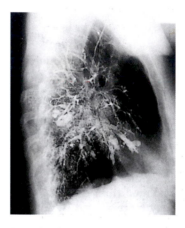

Bronchiectasis in a patient with allergic bronchopulmonary aspergillosis

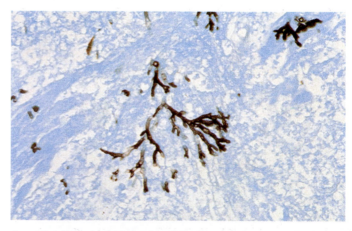

Aspergillus fumigatus hyphae and conidiophores (fruiting heads)

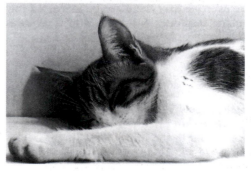

Cats are the most problematic domestic pet for asthmatics

Occupational asthma

The importance of occupational asthma is increasingly being recognised. Some estimates suggest that over 5% of cases of adult asthma have an occupational origin and over 200 precipitating agents have been reported. Asthmatic patients choosing a career should avoid occupations where they are likely to be exposed to large quantities of non-specific stimuli such as dust and cold air.

Definition

Occupational asthma is officially recognised as an industrial disease and subject to compensation. It is defined as asthma that "develops after a variable period of symptomless exposure to a sensitising agent at work." Fourteen agents are currently recognised for compensation and this list is kept under regular review. Agents such as proteolytic enzymes and laboratory animals are particularly likely to produce problems in atopic subjects, whereas isocyanate asthma is not related to atopic status. In some studies potent agents such as platinum salts have produced asthma in up to half of those who are exposed to them.

Diagnosis

Increased bronchial reactivity provoked by occupational agents may persist long after removal from exposure. Regular peak flow recordings are once again an important diagnostic tool and usually show a distinct relation to time at work, but the relationship may not be obvious because the timing of the responses is variable. Reactions may occur soon after arriving at work, be delayed until later in the day, or come on slowly over several days. In some cases a weekend away from work may not be long enough for lung function to return to normal and absence for a week or two may be necessary. Initial investigations include exploration of potential agents at work and recording peak flow patterns every two or four hours at and away from work. Further investigation may require specific challenge testing in an experienced laboratory.

Management

Awareness and early detection are important since occupational asthma is the one area where appropriate management can affect the natural history of the disease. The first approach to management should be to try to adjust the conditions at work that produced the sensitisation. If this is not possible the patient may be able to continue working with a mask to provide filtered air. If these measures fail and simple inhaled treatment is inadequate then a change of job will be necessary. It is advisable to try to obtain, with the patient's consent, the co-operation of any occupational health staff in the firm.

Within industry, problems arise most often from exposure to glutaraldehyde used in disinfection procedures, latex from gloves and proteins in the urine of small animals in laboratory technicians and researchers.

Food allergy

Food allergy causes eczema and gastrointestinal symptoms more often than asthma, but some striking cases do occur. Exclusion diets have generally given disappointing results in asthma; immediate skin prick tests and radioallergosorbent

Some causes of occupational asthma

Chemicals
  Isocyanates
  Platinum salts
  Epoxy resins
  Aluminium
  Hair sprays
  Azodicarbonamide (plastic blowing)

Vegetable sources
  Wood dusts
  Grains
  Coffee beans
  Colophony (solders)
  Cotton, flax, hemp dust
  Castor bean dust
  Latex

Enzymes
  Trypsin
  Bacillus subtilis

Animals
  Laboratory rodents
  Larger mammals
  Shellfish
  Locusts
  Grain weevil, mites

Drug manufacture
  Penicillins
  Piperazine
  Salbutamol
  Cimetidine
  Ispaghula
  Ipecacuanha

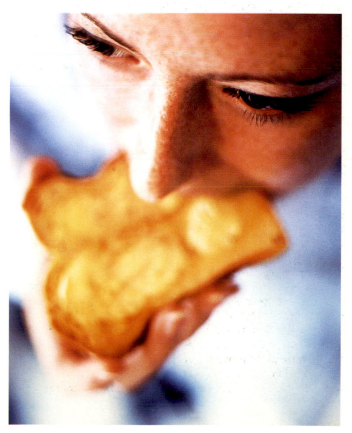

Food allergy is sometimes a factor in asthma Photo: Tony Stone Images

tests are less useful than for inhaled allergens. Most serious cases of asthma induced by food intolerance are evident from a carefully taken history, so elaborate diets are not warranted. When there is doubt, suspicions can be confirmed by excluding the agent from the diet or by controlled exposure.

Intolerance to food does not always indicate an allergic mechanism. Reactions may be related to pharmacological mediators such as histamine or tyramine in the food. They may be produced by food additives such as the yellow dye tartrazine, which is added to a wide range of foods and medications. When there is a specific allergy to foodstuffs, the most likely to be implicated are milk, eggs, nuts, and wheat.

Drug-induced asthma

Two main groups of drugs are responsible for most cases of drug-induced asthma: β-blocking agents and prostaglandin synthetase inhibitors such as aspirin.

β-blockers

β-blocking agents usually induce bronchoconstriction when given to asthmatic patients and this may happen even when they are given in eye drops. Relatively selective β-blockers such as atenolol and metoprolol are less likely to cause severe irreversible asthma, but the whole group of β-blocking drugs should be avoided in patients who already have asthma. For hypertension diuretics, angiotensin-converting enzyme inhibitors, or calcium antagonists are suitable alternatives. Calcium antagonists can also be used for angina and may even be beneficial in partially blocking exercise-induced asthma. When asthma is produced by β-blockade, large doses of β-stimulants are necessary to reverse it, particularly with less selective β-blockers. Fortunately, cardiac side-effects of treatment with β-stimulants are not a problem because they are also inhibited by the β-blockade.

Prostaglandin synthetase inhibitors

Salicylates provoke severe narrowing of the airways in a small group of adults with asthma. Once such a reaction has been noted these patients should avoid contact with aspirin or non-steroidal anti-inflammatory agents, which usually produce the same effects. The mechanism is probably related to changes in arachidonic acid metabolism with increased production of leukotrienes. Milder salicylate sensitivity can be shown more often on routine testing, particularly in adults with asthma and nasal polyps.

Ibuprofen is available without prescription and has the same effects. Patients are often unaware of the presence of salicylate in common compound preparations and cold cures. When salicylate sensitivity is suspected the patient should be asked to check carefully the contents of any such medication they take. When salicylate reactions occur it may be possible to induce tolerance by carefully building up from small oral doses. This should be done only in experienced units.

Iatrogenic effects

Occasionally drugs used to treat asthma can themselves be responsible for provoking bronchoconstriction. Such paradoxical effects have been described with aminophylline, ipratropium bromide, sodium cromoglycate, β-agonists in infants and propellants or contaminants from the valve apparatus in metered dose inhalers.

Drugs that can induce asthma
- β-blockers (including eye drops)
- Aspirin and non-steroidal anti-inflammatory drugs
- Inhaled asthma drugs
- Nebuliser solutions, hypotonic or with preservatives
- Angiotensin converting enzyme inhibitors

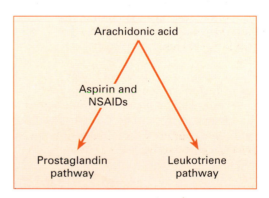

Aspirin blocks prostaglandin synthetase activity and sends arachidonic acid metabolism down the leukotriene pathway. This is likely to be the basis of aspirin-induced asthma

Hypotonic solutions are a potent cause of bronchoconstriction in people with asthma, and nebuliser solutions must always be made up with normal saline rather than water. Preservatives in some nebuliser solutions have also produced narrowing of the airways.

Emotional factors

Psychological factors can play an important part in asthma. On their own they do not produce asthma in subjects without an underlying susceptibility, but in the laboratory emotional factors and expectation can influence the bronchoconstrictor responses to various specific and non-specific stimuli and the bronchodilator responses to treatment. Stress and emotional disturbance are factors that must be taken into account in the overall management of asthmatic patients. In children the position is complicated by the emotional responses of their parents.

Confidence and relaxation

Emotional problems are more likely to occur when control of asthma is poor, and these problems are best managed by increasing the confidence of patients and relatives with adequate explanation and control of the asthma. It is particularly important that patients know exactly what to do during an acute exacerbation. More specific measures such as relaxation, yoga, hypnotherapy, and acupuncture have been investigated. Some trials have shown beneficial effects and some patients obtain considerable help from relaxation treatment. If conventional medicines are neglected when alternative approaches are adopted, however, it can be dangerous.

Asthma associated with emotional outbursts such as laughing and crying may be related to the response of the hyper-reactive airways to deep inspirations or to inhalation of cold, dry air rather than to the emotion itself. Manipulative patients may, of course, use a disease such as asthma for their own purposes just as they might use any other chronic disease.

Pollution

Personal air pollution with cigarette smoke worsens asthma; active and passive smoking provoke narrowing of the airways.

Air quality

There has been increased interest in environmental pollution in recent years. Though the inner city smogs disappeared after the introduction of the Clean Air Act 1956, high levels of ozone, sulphur dioxide, oxides of nitrogen, and particulate matter develop in certain areas and in particular climatic conditions. Combinations of high temperature, humidity, and heavy traffic can cause levels of these pollutants that are above the recommended guidelines of the World Health Organization. Increased symptoms and admissions have been linked to levels of nitrogen dioxide and sulphur dioxide – and, in some studies, ozone. High levels of small particulate matter are associated with increased mortality from cardio-respiratory diseases. Asthmatics should be aware of measures of air

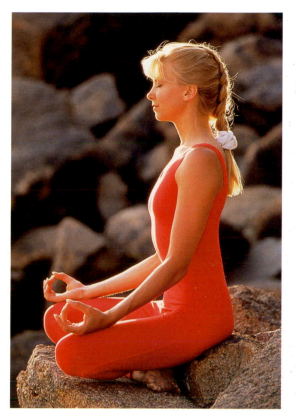

Relaxation can be of help, but is not a substitute for drug therapy Photo: The Stock Market

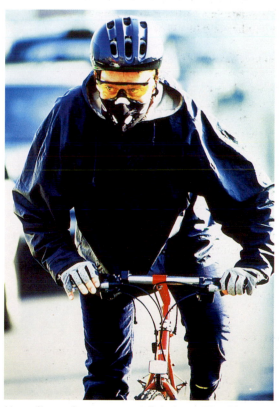

Air quality can be poor, especially in large cities Photo: Tony Stone Images

quality, and whenever possible they should keep away from areas of high pollution, particularly when exercising.

Weather
Climatic conditions such as the pressure and humidity associated with thunderstorms can provoke asthma. The conditions may increase the concentrations of fungal and pollen spores at ground level as they are brought down from higher levels of the atmosphere. The spores rupture to produce particles of respirable size.

Nitrogen dioxide
Levels of nitrogen dioxide found in the home may increase airway responses to common allergens such as house dust mite, and the average United Kingdom citizen spends 85 to 90% of their time indoors.

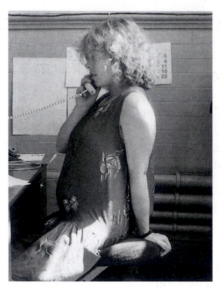

Women are naturally anxious about using drugs during pregnancy Photo: John Rae

Asthma and pregnancy

The control of asthma during pregnancy can change but the effect is variable. About a third of patients improve, a third worsen, and a third continue unchanged. The effect may vary in different pregnancies in the same woman. Breathlessness may be more pronounced in late pregnancy as the diaphragmatic movement is limited even without any change in airflow obstruction.

Drug treatment during pregnancy
There is a natural anxiety about the use of drugs during pregnancy. Fortunately the usual asthma treatments of inhaled β-antagonists, and inhaled and oral corticosteroids have been shown to be safe. Asthma control and supervision should be improved during pregnancy to reduce the likelihood of an acute exacerbation. Acute attacks should be treated vigorously in the normal way. Severe asthma and hypoxia rather than asthma treatments are the potential danger during pregnancy.

6 General management of acute asthma

Assessment of severity

The speed of onset of acute attacks varies. Some severe episodes come on over a period of minutes with no warning, although more often there is a background of deterioration over days or weeks. This period during which control of the asthma deteriorates tends to be longer in older patients. A good early guide to developing problems is the need to use bronchodilator inhalers more often than usual, or finding that they are less effective.

Peak flow monitoring

Deterioration in control can also be detected by regular monitoring of peak flow at home; a drop in the peak flow, or an increase in the diurnal variation of peak flow, provides evidence of instability. Detecting these changes allows a change of treatment while the decline is slow and before severe problems arise. All asthmatic patients should be aware of what to do if they fail to get relief from their usual treatment. A written action plan should be available for patients and relatives, which should include trigger levels of peak flow or symptoms that require changes in treatment or consultation for further advice.

Breathlessness

The most common symptom is breathlessness, and there is more likely to be a sensation of difficulty in inspiration than in expiration. Some patients have a poor appreciation of changes in the degree of their airflow obstruction and will complain of few symptoms until they have developed moderately severe asthma. They are more likely to develop severe asthma and are at particular risk during acute attacks. This is a group in which regular peak flow monitoring is particularly important.

Some studies of patients who have had life-threatening asthma show that patients with psycho-social problems, poor adherence to therapy and high levels of denial are over represented compared with control asthmatics.

As the severity of the asthma increases breathlessness begins to interfere with simple functions. Exercise is limited and later, eating and drinking are difficult. In severe attacks it will be difficult for the patient to speak in full sentences without gasping for breath between words. A knowledge of the pattern of previous attacks is important as the progress is often broadly similar in subsequent episodes.

Patients must be taught to seek help early rather than late in an acute exacerbation; it is easier to step in and prevent deterioration into severe asthma than to treat a full-blown attack. Patients and their families should all be confident about the management of exacerbations – not only their immediate treatment but seeking further help and hospital admission. These should all be discussed before the first acute attack of asthma.

Examination

Inability to speak will be obvious when taking the history. Respiratory rate is a useful sign and should be counted accurately; a rate of 25 beats per minute or above is a sign of

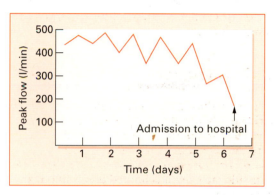

Gradual deterioration in peak flow in an acute exacerbation

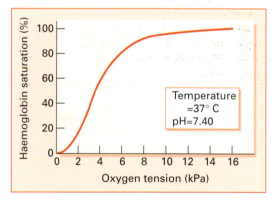

Normal oxyhaemoglobin dissociation curve. Saturation low enough to produce visible cyanosis is a sign of very severe asthma

severity. Hypoxia severe enough to cause confusion occurs only in severe asthma and means that admission to hospital and supplemental oxygen are needed urgently. The pulse rate is also a useful guide to severity: tachycardia over 110 beats per minute is found in severe episodes although this sign may be less reliable in the elderly when pulse rates tend to remain low. In very severe attacks bradycardia may occur.

Pulsus paradoxus (a drop in systolic pressure of more than 10 mm Hg on inspiration) is a traditional measurement in acute asthma. A drop of over 20 mm Hg is a sign of severe asthma, and changes correlate with progress and can be one way to monitor the effects of treatment. However, it is not always present even in severe asthma and is not routinely measured in many units. Any evidence of circulatory embarrassment, such as hypotension, is an indication for admission to hospital.

Chest sounds
Examination of the chest itself shows a fast respiratory rate, over-inflation, and wheezing. In very severe acute asthma airflow may be too little for an audible wheeze, so a quiet chest during an acute attack is worrying rather than reassuring. It may also indicate a pneumothorax (although these are not common in acute asthma, they are difficult to diagnose clinically; a chest X-ray film must be taken if there is any doubt).

Peak flow readings
In severe attacks the peak flow rate may be unrecordable. Peak flow or FEV_1 should be monitored throughout the attack and during recovery as they are reliable, simple guides to the effectiveness of treatment. Peak flow values are easier to interpret if the patient's usual or best readings are known.

Blood gases
An initial measurement of blood gases should be done in patients with asthma severe enough to warrant admission to hospital. Great care should be taken with blood gas measurements because some asthmatic patients who have had bad experiences of arterial puncture may delay attendance at hospital because of the memories of pain. In patients with mild attacks a pulse oximeter should be used in the accident and emergency department. If saturation is 93% or above while breathing air, and the patient does not have signs of severe asthma, then blood gas measurement can be omitted. In more severe cases oxygen saturation by pulse oximeter can be used to assess progress after the first arterial gas measurement, provided the initial carbon dioxide tension was not raised and there is no sign of appreciable deterioration.

Hypoxia and hypercapnia
Some hypoxia is usual and responds to supplemental oxygen. An arterial oxygen tension of less than 8kPa on air is a mark of severity. As long as the patient does not have COPD there is no need to limit the concentration of supplemental oxygen. The arterial carbon dioxide tension is usually low in acute asthma; occasionally, particularly in children, it is high on admission, but quickly responds to treatment with a bronchodilator. However, hypercapnia is an alarming feature of acute asthma and failure either to reduce carbon dioxide retention during the first hour, or to prevent its development during treatment, is an indication

that mechanical ventilation must be considered. The final decision on this depends on the overall clinical state of the patient rather than on the blood gas measurement alone.

Where to treat acute asthma

An acute attack of asthma is frightening; transfer to hospital might exacerbate symptoms by producing anxiety, and reassurance that treatment is available to relieve the attack is an important part of the management. It is not possible to lay down strict criteria for admission to hospital. The features of severity discussed above should, however, be assessed.

Most of the dangers of acute asthma come from a failure to appreciate the severity of an attack and the absence of suitable supervision and treatment to follow up the initial response. Immediate improvement after the first nebuliser treatment may provide false reassurance, being followed quickly by the return of severe asthma, so continued observation is essential.

Initial treatment
It may be obvious on first seeing the patient that supplemental oxygen and hospital treatment are necessary. Treatment should be started while this is arranged. In less severe attacks initial treatment should be given and, if the response is inadequate, hospital admission should be arranged. If the initial response is adequate it may be possible to manage the patient at home if supervision is available. The primary treatment should then be followed up, usually by adequate bronchodilation and corticosteroids, and the response should be assessed by measurements of peak flow. Threshold for admission should be lowered if there has been a recent admission, previous severe attacks, poor patient perception of severity or poor social support.

Dangers of under-treatment
Most deaths from asthma occur when the patient or doctor has failed to appreciate the severity of the attack. When there is any doubt it is safer to opt for vigorous treatment and admission to hospital. When treatment is given at home, the patient's condition must be assessed regularly and often until the exacerbation has settled. The reason for the acute exacerbation must then be sought.

Indications for immediate transfer to hospital
Signs
- Cyanosis, silent chest, poor respiratory effort
- Fatigue or exhaustion
- Agitation or reduced level of consciousness
- Difficulty in speaking
- *Pulsus paradoxus* >20 mm Hg
- Peak flow rate <25% of predicted

Response
- No improvement despite adequate doses of inhaled bronchodilator

---

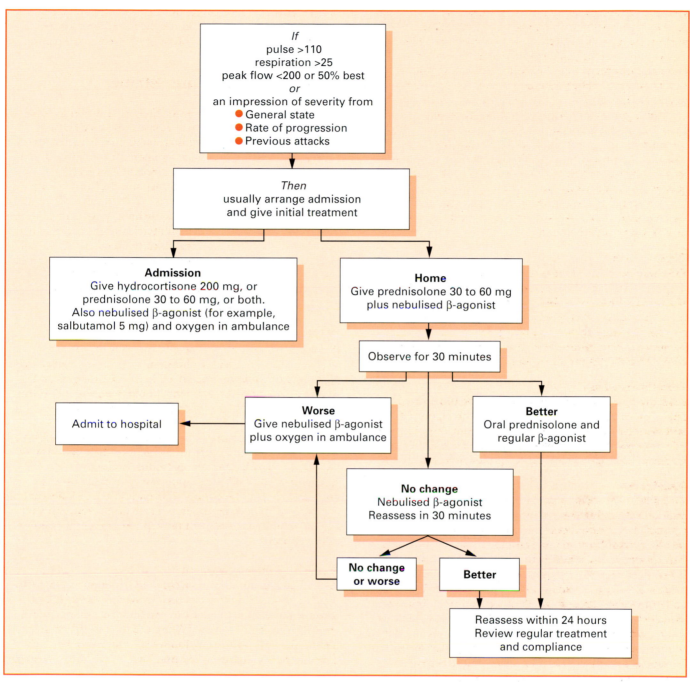

Treatment of acute severe asthma in general practice

7 Treatment of acute asthma

Introduction

The initial assessment of a patient with increased symptoms of asthma is very important. Most problems result from under-treatment and failure to appreciate severity. Monitor the peak flow rate and other signs before and after the first nebuliser treatment, and then as appropriate. In hospital, peak flow should be monitored at least four times daily for the duration of the stay. A flow chart for the management of asthma at home is shown in chapter 6 and a flow chart for management in hospital is shown later in this chapter. The various aspects of treatment are considered individually in this chapter.

β-stimulants

Adrenaline has been used in the treatment of asthma since just after the First World War. The specific β$_2$-stimulants such as salbutamol and terbutaline have replaced the earlier non-selective preparations for regular and acute use. There are no great differences in practice between the commonly used agents.

Use and availability of nebulisers

In acute asthma, metered dose inhalers often lose their effectiveness. This is largely because of difficulties in the delivery of the drugs to the airways and an alternative method of giving them is necessary – usually by nebuliser or intravenously. An alternative if a nebuliser is not available is a large volume spacer (Nebuhaler or Volumatic). Like the nebuliser it has the advantage of removing the need to co-ordinate inhaler actuation and breathing. There is little or no difference in the effectiveness of drugs that are nebulised or given intravenously in acute severe asthma, so nebulisation is generally preferable.

It is helpful for general practitioners to have nebulisers available for acute asthmatic attacks. β-stimulants are best given by nebulisers driven by oxygen in acute asthma, as they may even worsen hypoxia slightly through an effect on the pulmonary vasculature. In general practice the use of oxygen as the driving gas is not usually practical. Domiciliary oxygen sets do not produce a flow rate adequate to drive most nebulisers, but if available they can be used with nasal spectacles during the nebulisation for a patient having an acute attack. Many ambulance services are able to give nebulised drugs and oxygen during transfer to hospital.

In hospital, nebulisers used to treat asthmatic patients should be driven by oxygen except if the patient has COPD with carbon dioxide retention. The driving gas, flow rate, drug, diluent and volume of fill should be clearly written on the prescription chart. Dilutions should always be done with saline to avoid bronchoconstriction from nebulisation of hypotonic solutions. There is no real advantage of nebulisation with a machine capable of producing intermittent positive pressure.

For adults the initial dose should be 5 mg salbutamol or its equivalent. This should be halved if the patient has ischaemic heart disease. It is essential to continue the intensive treatment after the first response; many of the

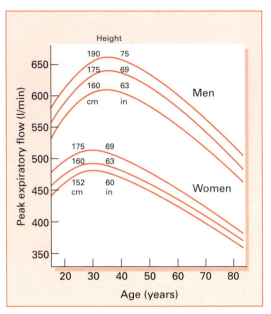

Peak expiratory flow in normal adults (Gregg I *et al*, *BMJ* 1989;**298**:1068–70)

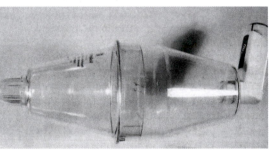

Attaching a volumatic spacer to a metered dose inhaler avoids the need for co-ordination between firing and inhalation

When a patient with acute asthma needs transfer to hospital from home, oral or intravenous steroids should be given before transfer

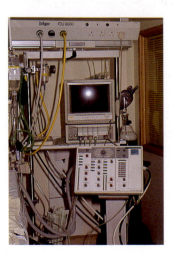

Acute attacks may require admission to the ITU

problems in acute asthma arise because of complacency after the initial response to the first treatment. In severe attacks the nebulisation may need to be repeated every 15 to 30 minutes and can even be continuous.

Parenteral delivery

If nebulised drugs are not effective then parenteral treatment should be considered. A reasonable plan is to give a β_2-agonist the first time, combine with an anticholinergic drug for the second nebulisation and move to intravenous bronchodilators if there is no improvement. If life-threatening features such as a raised carbon dioxide tension, an arterial oxygen tension less than 8kPa on oxygen, or a low pH are present, the intravenous agent should be used from the start.

The bronchodilator given parenterally in an acute attack can be β_2-agonist or aminophylline. There is little to choose between them. If the patient has been on theophylline and a level is not immediately available it is safer to use the β_2-stimulant. Salbutamol or terbutaline can be given intravenously over 10 minutes, or as an infusion, usually at 5 to 15 micrograms per minute. The adverse effects of tachycardia and tremor are much more common after intravenous injection than after nebulisation.

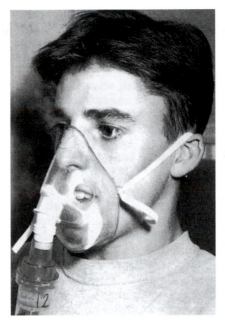

In acute asthma β-stimulants should be given by oxygen driven nebuliser

Anticholinergic agents

Ipratropium bromide is the only anticholinergic agent available in nebulised form in the United Kingdom. Nebulised ipratropium seems to be as effective as a nebulised β_2-stimulant in acute asthma. The dose of ipratropium is 500 micrograms and there are no problems with increased viscosity of secretions or mucociliary clearance at such doses. Ipratropium starts working more slowly than salbutamol: the peak response may not occur for 30 to 60 minutes.

Adverse reactions such as paradoxical bronchoconstriction have been reported occasionally. These were related mainly to the osmolality of the solution or to the preservatives and they have been corrected in the current preparations.

Although the combination of β-stimulant and anticholinergic agents produces a greater effect than use of a single agent, the difference is small and β-stimulants are sufficient for most patients. It is reasonable to start with a β-agonist alone and add ipratropium if the response to the first nebulisation is not considered adequate. If the initial assessment indicates that it is a very severe attack then the combination should be used from the start.

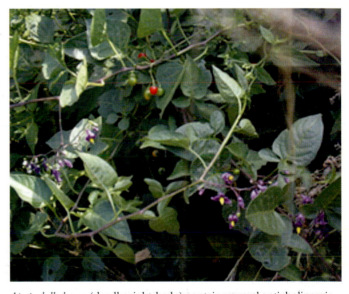

Atropa belladonna (deadly nightshade) contains several anticholinergic substances Photo: Science U.com

Methylxanthines

Aminophylline is an effective bronchodilator in acute asthma but most studies have shown that it is no more effective than a β-stimulant given by nebulisation or intravenously. There are more problems with its use than with nebulised drugs and it should be reserved for patients with life-threatening features or who have failed to respond to nebulised drugs. Toxic effects are common and can occur with drug concentrations in or just above the therapeutic range. Concentrations are difficult to predict from the dose given because of individual differences in metabolic rate and interactions with drugs such as nicotine, cimetidine, erythromycin and ciprofloxacin.

Theophylline clearance is reduced by:

- Erythromycin
- Cimetidine
- Allopurinol
- Frusemide
- Oral contraceptives
- Influenza vaccine
- Ciprofloxacin

The position is further complicated if patients are already taking oral theophyllines. The usual starting dose for intravenous aminophylline is 250 mg given over 20 to 30 minutes. If the patient has taken oral theophylline or aminophylline in the previous 24 hours and a blood concentration is not available then the initial dose should be omitted or halved. A continuous infusion is then given at a rate of 0.5 mg/kg/hour, though this dose should be reduced if the patient also has kidney or liver disease. If intravenous treatment is necessary for more than 24 hours then blood concentrations should be measured and the rate adjusted as necessary.

Corticosteroids

Corticosteroids are effective in preventing the development of acute asthma.

Oral delivery

Oral prednisolone should be given if control of asthma is deteriorating despite adequate bronchodilator treatment. A single oral dose of prednisolone, 20 to 40 mg according to body weight, should be given each day for 7 to 14 days according to the speed of the response. The dose may then be stopped abruptly. If this opportunity is missed and an acute attack of asthma does develop corticosteroids are still an important element in treatment. Fatal attacks of asthma are associated with failure to prescribe any or adequate doses of corticosteroids. No noticeable response occurs for four to six hours, so corticosteroids should be started as early as possible and intensive bronchodilator treatment used while waiting for them to take effect.

Intravenous delivery

In most cases oral corticosteroids are adequate, but when there are life-threatening features intravenous hydrocortisone should be used in an initial dose of 200 mg followed by 200 mg six hourly for 24 hours. Prednisolone should be started at a dose of 30 to 60 mg daily, whether or not hydrocortisone is used (50 mg prednisolone is equivalent to 200 mg hydrocortisone). If the patient is first seen at home and transferred to hospital the first dose of corticosteroid should be given together with initial bronchodilator treatment before leaving home.

Length of steroid course

When intensive initial treatment has been required prednisolone should be maintained at a dose of 30 mg per day for at least a week. Two to three weeks of treatment may be needed to obtain the maximal response with deflation to normal lung volumes and loss of excessive diurnal variations of peak flow. There are few side-effects of such short courses of corticosteroids. Increased appetite, fluid retention, gastrointestinal upset and psychological disturbance are the most common. Exposure to *Herpes zoster* may produce severe infections in susceptible individuals.

Oxygen

Acute severe asthma is always associated with hypoxia, although cyanosis develops late and is a grave sign. Death in asthma is caused by severe hypoxia; oxygen should be given as soon as possible. It is very unusual to provoke carbon

Airway responses to oral and intravenous corticosteroids take place slowly, over several hours

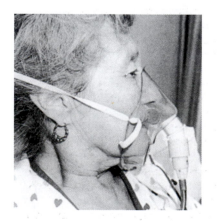

Nebulisers should ideally be oxygen driven

dioxide retention with oxygen treatment in asthma, so oxygen should be given freely during transfer to hospital where blood gas measurement can be made. Masks can provide 40 to 50% oxygen.

Nebulisers should be driven by oxygen whenever possible. In older subjects with an exacerbation of COPD there is a potential danger of carbon dioxide retention. In these cases treatment should begin with 24% or 28% oxygen by Venturi mask until the results of blood gas measurements are available.

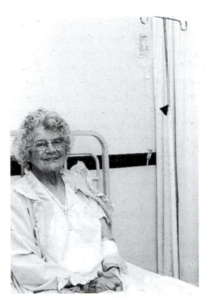

Fluid and electrolytes

Patients with acute asthma tend to be dehydrated because they are often too breathless to drink and because fluid loss from the respiratory tract is increased. Dehydration increases the viscosity of mucus, making plugging of the airways more likely, so intravenous fluid replacement is often necessary. Three litres should be given during the first 24 hours if little oral fluid is being taken.

Some patients admitted to hospital with an acute attack will need intravenous rehydration

Potassium supplements
Increased alveolar ventilation, sympathomimetic drugs and corticosteroids all tend to lower the serum potassium concentration. This is the most common disturbance of electrolytes in acute asthma; the serum potassium concentration should be monitored and supplements given as necessary.

Antibiotics

Upper respiratory tract infections are the most common trigger factors for acute asthma and most of these are viral. In only a few cases are exacerbations of asthma precipitated by bacterial infection.

Antibiotics should be reserved for patients who have evidence of infection

There is no evidence of benefit from the routine use of antibiotics. They should be reserved for patients in whom there is presumptive evidence of infection – such as fever, neutrophils in the blood or sputum, or radiological changes. Although all these features may occur in acute attacks without bacterial infection, an antibiotic such as amoxycillin or erythromycin would be appropriate.

Controlled ventilation

Patients with acute severe asthma who need hospital admission should be treated in an area able to deal with acute medical emergencies, with adequate nursing and medical supervision. If hypoxia is worsening, hypercapnia is present, or patients are exhausted or drowsy, then they should be nursed in an intensive care unit.

Occasionally, mechanical ventilation may be necessary for a short time while the treatment takes effect. It is usually needed because the patient becomes exhausted; experience and careful observation are necessary to judge the right time to begin ventilatory support. It can sometimes be avoided by the use of inspiratory positive airway pressure through a close fitting face mask, but patients may find it difficult to tolerate this treatment.

High inflation pressures and long expiratory times may make ventilation difficult in asthmatic patients, but most

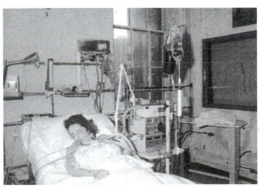

Mechanical ventilation is sometimes necessary in acute severe asthma

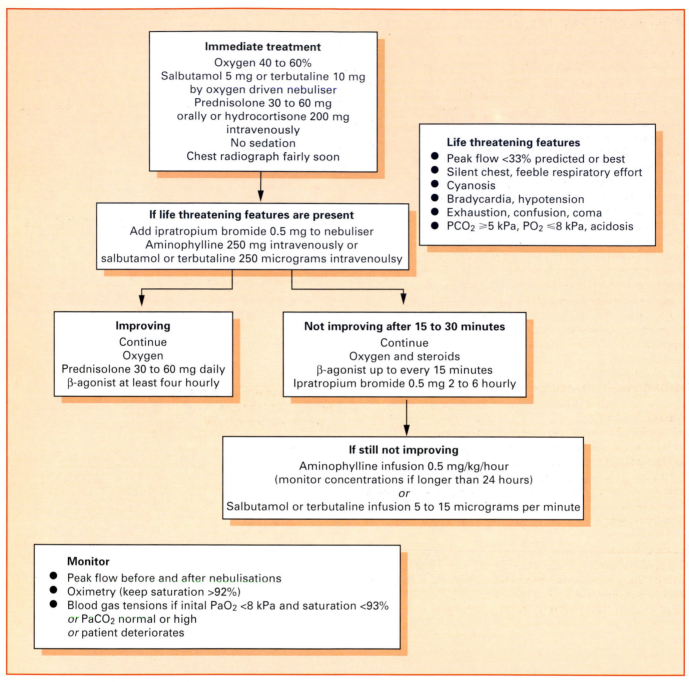

Immediate treatment
Oxygen 40 to 60%
Salbutamol 5 mg or terbutaline 10 mg
by oxygen driven nebuliser
Prednisolone 30 to 60 mg
orally or hydrocortisone 200 mg
intravenously
No sedation
Chest radiograph fairly soon

Life threatening features
- Peak flow <33% predicted or best
- Silent chest, feeble respiratory effort
- Cyanosis
- Bradycardia, hypotension
- Exhaustion, confusion, coma
- $PCO_2 \geqslant 5$ kPa, $PO_2 \leqslant 8$ kPa, acidosis

If life threatening features are present
Add ipratropium bromide 0.5 mg to nebuliser
Aminophylline 250 mg intravenously or
salbutamol or terbutaline 250 micrograms intravenoulsy

Improving
Continue
Oxygen
Prednisolone 30 to 60 mg daily
β-agonist at least four hourly

Not improving after 15 to 30 minutes
Continue
Oxygen and steroids
β-agonist up to every 15 minutes
Ipratropium bromide 0.5 mg 2 to 6 hourly

If still not improving
Aminophylline infusion 0.5 mg/kg/hour
(monitor concentrations if longer than 24 hours)
or
Salbutamol or terbutaline infusion 5 to 15 micrograms per minute

Monitor
- Peak flow before and after nebulisations
- Oximetry (keep saturation >92%)
- Blood gas tensions if inital PaO_2 <8 kPa and saturation <93%
  or $PaCO_2$ normal or high
  or patient deteriorates

Treatment of acute severe asthma in hospital

experienced units have good results provided that the decision to ventilate the patient is made electively and is not precipitated by respiratory arrest. When patients being mechanically ventilated fail to improve on adequate treatment, bronchial lavage may occasionally be considered to reopen airways that have become plugged by mucus. In very severe unresponsive cases other treatments such as inhalational anaesthetics may be helpful, or a mixture of helium and oxygen may improve airflow while other treatment takes effect.

Other factors

Most patients with acute severe asthma improve with these measures. Occasionally physiotherapy may be useful to help patients cough up thick plugs of sputum, but mucolytic agents to change the nature of the secretions do not help.

An episode of asthma is frightening. The dangerous use of sedatives such as morphine was common before effective treatment became available. Unfortunately this practice still continues, with occasional fatal consequences. Treatment of agitation should be aimed at reversing the asthma precipitating it, not at producing respiratory depression.

Discharge from hospital

Discharge too early is associated with increased readmission and with mortality. Patients should have stopped nebuliser treatment and be using their own inhalers, with the proper technique checked, for at least 24 hours before discharge. Ideally peak flow should be above 75% of the patient's predicted or best known reading. Diurnal variability should be below 25%.

A few patients may never lose their morning dips and may have to be discharged with them still present. For every patient the reason for the acute episode should be sought and appropriate changes made in their routine treatment and in their response to any deterioration in an attempt to avoid similar attacks in the future. Patients with an acute attack of asthma should be looked after or at least seen by a physician with an interest in respiratory disease during their inpatient stay. Follow up should be arranged and a respiratory specialist nurse will be helpful in education, management and support.

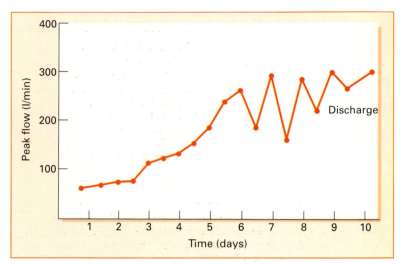

Peak flow during recovery from acute attack

Subsequent management

Patients should not be discharged from hospital until their asthma is stable on the treatment that they will take at home. They should leave with a plan of further management. This should include peak flow monitoring and a plan to respond to deterioration in the control of their asthma. The general practitioner should be informed of the admission and the subsequent plans, and should see the patient within a week.

Good communication between the hospital and the general practitioner is essential

Hospital follow-up
The patient should return to the chest clinic within a month. Good communication between hospital and general practitioner is vital around this vulnerable period – telephone, fax and electronic links may help.

8　General management of chronic asthma

Guidelines

Various guidelines have been produced and published for the management of asthma. In the United Kingdom those produced by the British Thoracic Society, National Asthma Campaign and Royal College of Physicians in association with accident and emergency, primary care and paediatric groups have had wide distribution and acceptance. The 1995 review and position statement was published in early 1997.[1] A further revision with a clear evidence base is being produced. In chronic asthma the guidelines define a number of steps or levels of treatment.

Initially there was a perception that patients should work up through the steps until control was achieved. The latest version makes it clear that entry should be at a step likely to gain control with subsequent reduction when stable.

Guidelines are most likely to influence behaviour when they are adapted to local needs in hospital or practice and endorsed by a local respected enthusiast. They should be accompanied by regular audit against the agreed parts of the guidelines.

Most of the published guidelines are in broad agreement on the strategy for managing chronic asthma.

The guidelines of the National Heart, Lung and Blood Institute (NHLBI) in the United States differentiate between mild intermittent, mild persistent, moderate persistent and severe persistent asthma. These relate to the first three steps and combined steps 4 and 5 of the BTS guidelines. The level of β-agonist use for progress to regular anti-inflammatory therapy varies, once daily for the BTS and over twice a week for the NHLBI

General features

As a preliminary step in all patients with asthma, obvious precipitating factors should be sought and avoided when practicable. This is possible for specific allergens such as animals and foods, but is not usually feasible with more widespread allergens such as pollens and house dust mites. A common non-specific stimulus is cigarette smoking. Up to a fifth of asthmatics continue to smoke; strenuous efforts should be made to discourage smoking in asthmatic patients and their families. Precipitating factors should be carefully explored on one of the first visits but they should also be reassessed periodically.

Fortunately, most asthmatic patients can have their disease controlled by safe drug treatment, with minimal side-effects. Education of the patient in understanding the disease and treatment is often helped by home peak flow recording and written explanations of the purpose and practical details of treatment. In particular, the differences between symptomatic bronchodilator treatment and regular maintenance treatment must be emphasised. It is all too common to find asthmatic patients using their dose of inhaled steroid or sodium cromoglycate only to treat an acute attack. Trained nurses can be helpful in continuing education and supervision.

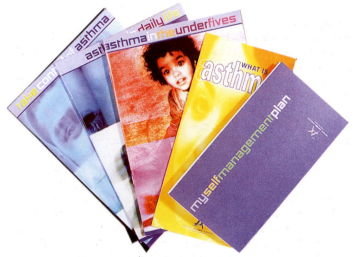

A selection of the educational leaflets produced by the National Asthma Campaign

Asthma clinics

Many hospitals have concentrated their patients into specific asthma clinics for some years. Many general practices have specific asthma or respiratory disease clinics run by practice nurses. Others use the nurses in clinics for other chronic conditions as well as asthma. Local and national training courses are available for nurses who take on such clinics. The clinics can be used to audit the treatment of asthmatic patients in a practice and to ensure that all patients are encouraged to participate in their optimal management.

Asthma clinics in general practice are best if they work with clearly written management guidelines and care plans. In some practices they are run by doctors, but in most cases they are run by nurses, who have more time to spend with each individual patient to go through inhaler techniques, understanding and management plans. An interested doctor should be available for consultation and a close liaison should be built up with chest physicians at the local hospital.

Aims of management

Persistent inflammation of the airways and increased bronchial reactivity have been recognised even in mild intermittent asthma. The inflammation can be targeted by drugs such as inhaled corticosteroids, which reduce bronchial hyper-responsiveness, symptoms and inflammatory infiltration of the airway. There has been a general move to be more aggressive in the treatment of asthma, the goal being freedom from symptoms rather than tolerance of shortness of breath and frequent need of bronchodilators.

Drug regimes

Routine regular use of bronchodilators should be avoided. They should be used to treat symptoms and their use should be limited by the use of prophylactic agents. This approach fits with the various sets of guidelines published over the last few years. Theophyllines probably leave airway reactivity unchanged and have not been associated with accelerated decline in lung function; there is renewed interest in their possible anti-inflammatory role. Some of these findings require confirmation.

Regular inhaled corticosteroids, however, decrease reactivity, as (probably) do sodium cromoglycate and nedocromil sodium. There is now evidence from studies of mild asthma that regular use of prophylactic agents reduces inflammation of the airways. The hope is that the reduction in the inflammation will prevent damage to the airway that would otherwise go on to produce irreversible obstruction. There is not yet any long-term evidence for this, nor is there convincing evidence that inhaled steroids change the natural history of asthma in any other way. Reactivity is improved but not returned to normal. Leukotriene receptor antagonists have also shown evidence of an anti-inflammatory action in addition to bronchodilatation.

Mild episodes of wheezing occurring once or twice a month can be controlled with inhaled β-stimulants. When attacks are more frequent regular treatment with inhaled steroids or sodium cromoglycate is necessary. Lack of

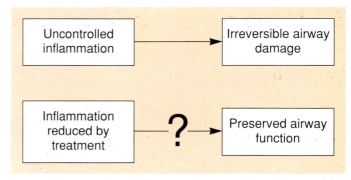

Aims of management of asthma

The ultimate goal is freedom from symptoms

The objectives of steps 1 to 3 adapted from the BTS guidelines are:

- No chronic symptoms
- Minimal exacerbations
- Minimal need for relief bronchodilators
- No limitations on activity, including exercise
- Circadian peak expiratory flow (PEF) variation greater than 20%
- PEF of 80% or over, predicted or best
- No adverse effects from treatment

At steps 4 to 5 such freedom from symptoms may not be achievable without side-effects and the objectives are:

- Fewest possible symptoms
- Least possible need for relief bronchodilators
- Least possible limitation of activity
- Least possible PEF variation
- Best PEF
- Fewest adverse effects from treatment

adequate control should be sought by questions about sensitivity to irritants such as dust and smoke, questions about night-time symptoms, and by peak flow recording. Definite diurnal variation on peak flow readings or nocturnal waking indicates a high degree of reactivity of the airways and the need for vigorous treatment.

When chronic symptoms persist in the face of appropriate inhaled treatment a short course of oral corticosteroids often produces improvement, which may last for many months after the course.

In a variable disease such as asthma, in which monitoring of the state of the disease is comparatively easy, the education and co-operation of the patient are vital parts of management. The patient should know how and when to take each treatment, broadly what each does and exactly what to do in an exacerbation.

Reference

1. *Thorax.* The British Guidelines on Asthma Management. 1995 Review and Position Statement. 1997;**52** suppl 1.

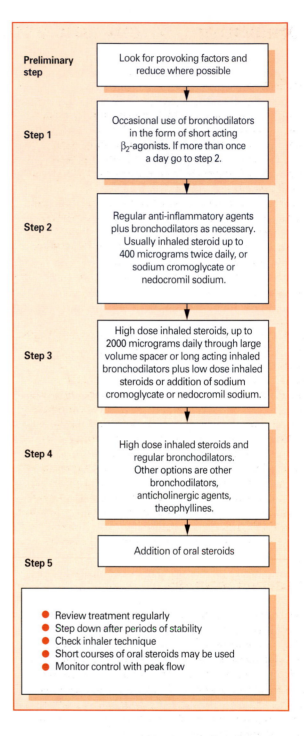

Stepwise treatment of asthma (adapted from the British Thoracic Society guidelines). The inhaled steroid would be beclomethasone dipropionate, budesonide or fluticasone propionate (starting at half the dose shown)

9 Treatment of chronic asthma

β-stimulants

The first line of treatment of mild intermittent asthma is one of the selective β_2-stimulants taken by inhalation. β-stimulants are the most effective bronchodilator in asthma. They start to work quickly – salbutamol and terbutaline take effect within 15 minutes and last for four to six hours. If more than one daily dose is usually required then additional treatment must be considered. The dose response varies among patients as does the dose that will produce side-effects, such as tremor. Patients should be taught to monitor their inhaler use and to understand that if they need it more, or if its effects lessen, these are danger signals. They indicate deterioration in asthmatic control and the need for further treatment.

Adverse effects
Some patients worry that β-stimulants may become slightly less effective with time, particularly if the dose is high. There is little evidence of appreciable tachyphylaxis for the airway effects in asthmatics. If it exists, it is a minor effect that is quickly reversed, either by stopping the treatment temporarily, or by taking corticosteroids. Tremor, palpitations and muscle cramps may occur, but are rarely troublesome if the drug is inhaled; these adverse effects outside the lung often become less of a problem with continued treatment.

Some studies found that regular use of β-stimulants was associated with increased bronchial reactivity, worsening asthma control and accelerated decline of lung function. These have not been confirmed and, in any case, when the steps in the BTS guidelines are followed, β-stimulants are not used regularly unless needed for control of symptoms.

Long acting β-agonists

The place of the long acting inhaled β-agonists salmeterol and eformoterol has been a matter of debate during the 1990s. The mechanism of the prolonged action is different with the two drugs and the onset of bronchodilatation is faster with eformoterol, but the two drugs are regarded as equivalent by most physicians. Choice between them is dependent more on the device required than the drug itself. They are particularly effective for nocturnal asthma and for exercise-induced asthma.

Several studies have shown that salmeterol is more effective than doubling inhaled corticosteroids in controlling symptoms and increasing peak flow. The effect is maintained over six months in such studies. A comparison of low and high-dose inhaled steroids over 12 months, with or without eformoterol, showed that increasing steroids and eformoterol reduced exacerbations. Severe exacerbations, defined by need for oral steroids or peak flow drop, were prevented more effectively by higher dose steroids than eformoterol, but best of all by the combination. Eformoterol added to steroids was the most effective in symptom reduction and peak flow control. It is important to remember that the long acting β-agonists are

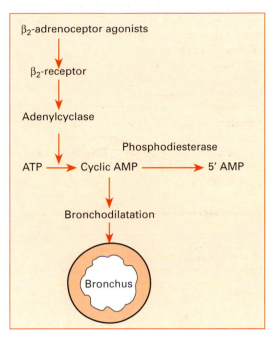

Increases in cyclic AMP lead to bronchodilatation and may be produced by β_2-receptor stimulation or phosphodiesterase inhibition

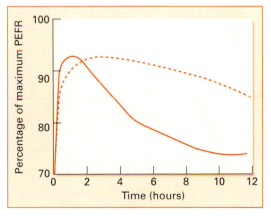

Bronchodilator response to oral salbutamol 200 micrograms (solid line) and inhaled salmeterol 50 micrograms (broken line) (Ullman A *et al*, *Thorax* 1988;**43**:674–8)

The information available suggests that when step 2 of the BTS guidelines has been reached and control needs to be improved, the best symptom control at step 3 is achieved by adding a long acting inhaled bronchodilator to low-dose inhaled steroid (for instance, 400 micrograms beclomethasone or budesonide daily). If the problem is peak flow instability and frequent exacerbations, then raising the inhaled steroid or combining the two approaches may be the best approach. Whatever the approach at step 3, the next step will normally be the combination of higher dose inhaled steroids and long acting inhaled β-agonists

bronchodilators and do not suppress inflammation. In asthma they should always be given in combination with inhaled steroids and the patient must not drop these on starting or finding a highly effective medication. In addition they should carry a short acting β-agonist to use for acute symptoms. Adverse effects of salmeterol and eformoterol are the same as those of short acting agents.

Anticholinergic bronchodilators

Ipratropium bromide blocks the cholinergic bronchoconstrictor effect of the vagus nerve. It is a non-selective antagonist blocking inhibitory M_2 receptors on postganglionic nerves as well as M_3 receptors on airway smooth muscle. Oxitropium bromide has a longer action, which makes it suitable for use two or three times a day and a longer acting agent tiotropium is likely to become available.

Effectiveness

Anticholinergics are most effective in very young children and in older patients. They are as effective or more effective than β-stimulants in COPD. In most cases of asthma, anticholinergic agents are less effective than β-stimulants, but they may supplement their effect if reversibility is incomplete. Anticholinergics take second place as bronchodilators in asthma unless tremor or tachycardia are troublesome side-effects.

If the response to a β-stimulant is inadequate then the technique of using the inhaler should be checked first. If this is satisfactory, evidence of an extra anticholinergic effect should be sought by measuring peak flow before and after inhalation of the β-agonist and then 30 to 60 minutes after adding the anticholinergic. At these doses there is no drying of secretions or interference with mucociliary clearance.

Methylxanthines

Theophylline is an effective bronchodilator and may also have anti-inflammatory actions. Its safety margin is low compared with other bronchodilators that can be given by inhalation. Individual differences in the doses required are high, so that it is necessary to monitor treatment by blood concentrations. Inhaled treatment with β-agonists is preferable, but slow release theophyllines are an alternative to long acting β-agonists for nocturnal symptoms. Absorption of aminophylline from suppositories is much less predictable and they are best avoided.

Adverse effects

The most common side-effects of theophylline are nausea, vomiting and abdominal discomfort, but headache, malaise, fast pulse rate and fits also occur, sometimes without early warning from gastrointestinal symptoms. The dose of theophylline should start at around 7 mg/kg/day in divided doses and should then be built up. All patients taking theophylline should have their serum concentrations monitored and doses adjusted until they are between 8 and 18 mg/l (40 to 90 micromol/l) for optimal bronchodilator effect. Above 20 mg/l toxic effects are unacceptably high, although 15% to 30% of patients will have gastrointestinal effects with smaller doses.

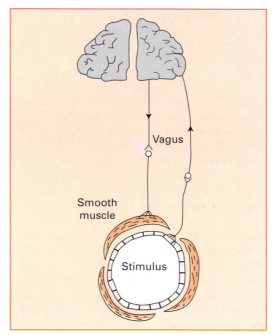

Anticholinergic agents block vagal efferent stimulation of bronchial smooth muscle

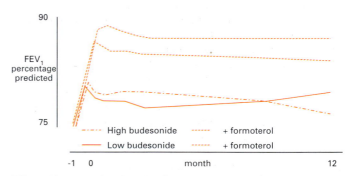

Effect of formoterol with and without a corticosteroid[1]

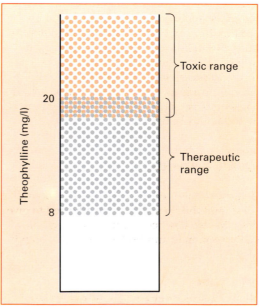

There is no safety margin between therapeutic and toxic ranges with theophylline

Theophylline clearance is increased by smoking, alcohol consumption and enzyme inducing drugs such as phenytoin, rifampicin and barbiturates. Clearance will be decreased and blood concentrations will rise if it is given at the same time as cimetidine, ciprofloxacin or erythromycin and in the presence of heart failure, liver impairment or pneumonia.

Lower theophylline levels, with a lower risk of side-effects, have been shown to have an anti-inflammatory effect *in vivo* and *in vitro*. This is a possible alternative, at drug levels of 5 to 15 mg/l, at steps 2 and 3 but more studies are needed before this can be regarded as a real alternative to inhaled steroids.

Mast cell stabilisers

Sodium cromoglycate

Sodium cromoglycate blocks bronchoconstrictor responses to challenge by exercise and antigens. The original proposed mechanism of stabilisation of mast cells may not be the main mechanism of its action in asthma. It can be used as the first-line prophylactic agent if control of asthma requires more than an occasional inhalation of β-agonist; success is most likely with young atopic asthmatic patients, but may occur at any age.

Sodium cromoglycate used to be given as a dry powder in Spincaps but metered dose inhalers delivering 5 mg per actuation are more convenient and just as effective. Occasionally patients develop reflex bronchoconstriction in response to the irritant effects of the dry powder; if they do, they should try changing to a metered dose inhaler or using a dose of inhaled β-agonist 10 to 15 minutes earlier. Other adverse reactions to sodium cromoglycate are rare.

Other mast cell stabilisers have been disappointing, possibly because of the additional effects of cromoglycate. The oral agent ketotifen produces drowsiness in 10% of patients and has little activity.

Cromoglycate should not be dismissed as ineffective until it has been tried for at least four to eight weeks and it must be used regularly. It has no place in the treatment of acute exacerbations of asthma.

Nedocromil sodium

Nedocromil sodium has the same properties as sodium cromoglycate but may have an additional anti-inflammatory effect on the airway epithelium and reduce coughing. It is probably more useful than sodium cromoglycate in older patients, although it is less effective than inhaled corticosteroids in most subjects. It may be tried as a first line in patients with mild disease, or as an addition to inhaled corticosteroids when control of symptoms is inadequate.

Inhaled corticosteroids

Steroids may be given by metered dose inhaler, dry powder devices or nebuliser and the dose should be adjusted to give optimum control. The two most common inhaled steroids, beclomethasone dipropionate and budesonide, are roughly equivalent in dose.

Method of delivery

The formulation and delivery device must be considered. The non-CFC beclomethasone metered dose inhaler QVar has a small particle size and increased lung deposition.

> Sodium cromoglycate must be used regularly for at least 4 to 8 weeks before being dismissed as ineffective

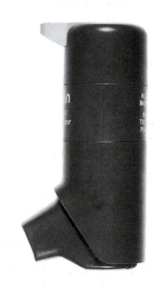

The Autohaler is triggered by inspiratory airflow. Breath-actuated metered dose inhalers are available for β-agonists, anticholinergics, cromoglycate, and corticosteroids

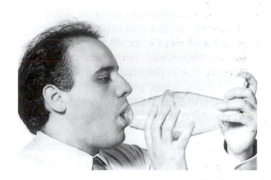

Large volume spacers overcome problems with co-ordination of inhaler firing and inspiration. They reduce oropharyngeal deposition of the aerosol and improve delivery to the lung

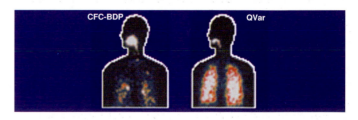

Deposition of beclomethasone dipropionate using a CFC-containing metered dose inhaler and the CFC-free QVar inhaler.[2] The latter produces a substantial increase in lung deposition Photo: 3M Healthcare

The dose of beclomethasone can be halved when switching from another preparation.

Fluticasone propionate
The newer agent fluticasone propionate can be used at half the dose of beclomethasone dipropionate with the same therapeutic effect and equivalent or reduced systemic effects. Much of the benefit of inhaled corticosteroids is seen at low to moderate doses, although there is a further effect with higher doses.

Adverse effects
In adults there are no problems, apart from occasional oropharyngeal candidiasis, or a husky voice, until a daily dose above the equivalent of 1000 micrograms beclomethasone dipropionate is reached. At higher doses there may be biochemical evidence of suppression of the hypothalamic-pituitary-adrenal axis, even with inhaled steroids. Much of the systemic effect comes from absorption from the lung itself, by-passing the metabolic pathways of the gut and liver that limit any problems from drug deposited in the mouth and swallowed.

With doses of more than 1000 micrograms daily of budesonide or beclomethasone there are metabolic effects, including an increase in the concentration of osteocalcin, a marker of increased bone turnover. There is some evidence of skin thinning and purpura, even in patients who have not had appreciable doses of oral steroids. Doses over 2000 micrograms daily are not often used but when necessary nebulised budesonide or fluticasone may be a convenient strategy. A large volume spacer should be used at doses above 800 micrograms daily to reduce the pharyngeal deposition of metered dose inhalers. At 1500 micrograms and above it is advisable for patients to carry a steroid card, especially if they use occasional courses of oral steroids.

Regular use
Doses of inhaled steroids should be taken regularly to be effective. Doubling the regular dose when an upper respiratory infection develops is often advised and may reduce the risk of problems from an exacerbation of asthma.

Compliance
The main difficulties in the use of inhaled corticosteroids are the patients' worries about the use of steroids and the difficulties of ensuring that patients take regular medication even when they are well. These problems are increased by the move to use inhaled corticosteroids earlier in asthma and to try to achieve a level of control that is free of symptoms. In mild asthma, under good control, once daily administration may be appropriate rather than the usual twice daily.

Dosage reduction
There is a suggestion that control is achieved more easily by the use of a high dose of inhaled steroids at the start, then a reduction as control is achieved. When asthma is under control the next decision is how long to maintain the inhaled steroids. The dose should be reviewed regularly and if doses above 1000 micromoles daily have been necessary these should be reduced when possible. Most physicians like to have complete asthma control for six to twelve months before trying to stop prophylaxis completely.

Side-effects of inhaled corticosteroids
Established:
Oropharyngeal candidiasis
Dysphonia
Irritation and cough
Purpura and thinning of skin
Cataracts

Suggested at high dose:
Adrenal suppression
Reduced growth in children
Osteoporosis

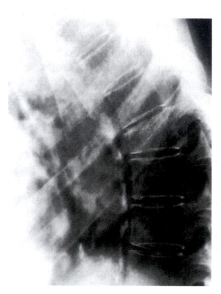

Osteoporotic collapse of a thoracic vertebra in a patient taking oral steroids

Oral corticosteroids

Occasional asthmatic patients have to take long-term oral corticosteroids but this should be only after the failure of vigorous treatment with other drugs. The symptoms or risks of the disease must be balanced against the adverse effects of long-term treatment with oral corticosteroids. It is important to remember that, in contrast, short courses of oral steroids for exacerbations of symptoms and inhaled steroids have few serious problems.

Length of treatment
Short courses of oral steroids may be stopped abruptly or tailed off over a few days. Low concentrations of cortisol and adrenocorticotrophic hormone (ACTH) are found for just two to three days after 40 mg prednisolone daily for three weeks, but clinical problems with responses to stress or exacerbations of asthma do not occur. An appropriate course would be 25 to 40 mg prednisolone daily for 14 days. Most asthmatic patients can be taught to keep such a supply of steroids at home and to use them according to their individual management plan when predetermined signs of deteriorating control occur.

If patients require long-term oral steroids, they should be settled on a regimen of treatment on alternate days whenever possible. The goal is always to establish control with other treatment that will allow the discontinuation of the oral steroids. Inhaled steroids in moderate to high doses should be maintained to keep the oral dose as low as possible. Alternative preparations such as ACTH and triamcinolone are less flexible and give no appreciable benefit in terms of adrenal suppression.

Resistance
A small proportion of asthmatic patients are fully or partially resistant to corticosteroids. They form a particularly difficult group to treat.

Adverse effects
When patients are on long-term oral steroids or take short courses more than three times a year the risks of osteoporosis should be considered. Bone density should be measured and if it starts low, or declines on treatment, biphosphonates should be considered. Other measures such as regular exercise, hormone replacement and calcium intake should be addressed in all patients on oral steroids.

Patients on steroids should be advised to avoid contact with chickenpox and *Herpes zoster* while on therapy and for three months after prolonged use.

Leukotriene antagonists

After many years of only minor changes to the standard drug classes, a new class of drugs has become available with the development of oral inhibitors of leukotriene production or action. Antagonists of cysteinyl leukotrienes (LTC4, LTD4 and LTE4) such as montelukast, pranlukast and zafirlukast act as selective competitive inhibitors of receptors on smooth muscle and elsewhere. Zileuton is a 5-lipoxygenase inhibitor reducing the production of leukotrienes from arachidonic acid in mast cells, eosinophils, and basophils.

Leukotrienes produce marked bronchoconstriction in addition to oedema, mucus secretion and reduced mucociliary clearance. These drugs have been found to block early and late responses to allergen challenge and to be effective in exercise and aspirin induced asthma. They have been shown to be useful in moderate persistent asthma as an addition to inhaled steroids. They are effective also in mild persistent asthma; zafirlukast and zileuton have been included at this point (step 2) in the 1997 NHLBI guidelines from the United States.

Adverse reactions
More work is needed on comparisons of leukotrienes with inhaled steroids as first-line anti-inflammatory agents. Drug interactions occur with zileuton. Zafirlukast has been associated with cases of Churg Strauss syndrome (allergic granulomatosis) in patients reducing oral steroids, but it seems likely that this was unmasked by steroid reduction rather than a drug effect. The drugs are generally well tolerated.

Steroid sparing agents

In patients requiring oral steroids to maintain control, a number of other agents have been used to try to reduce the steroid dose and avoid the associated side-effects. All these treatments have side-effects of their own and all other conventional therapies should be in place or tried before accepting that chronic oral steroid treatment is needed.

Methotrexate
There have been a number of trials of methotrexate, usually taken orally once a week. Around half of these have been positive with a significant reduction in steroid dose, and a trial of two to three months treatment may be appropriate in some patients. Adverse effects are on the bone marrow, liver and lung.

Other agents
Cyclosporin has been effective in several studies, producing some improvement in control with a small decrease in steroid dose. Renal toxicity is a problem with cyclosporin. Gold and colchicine have been tested in some studies but are not in regular use.

Desensitisation and avoidance of allergens

As discussed in chapter 5, the results of trials of desensitisation and avoidance of allergens have been disappointing. Some patients have obvious precipitating factors – in particular, animals – and avoidance is helpful, but there are usually other unknown precipitating factors. More common are patients with reactive airways who are also sensitive to pollens, house dust mite and other allergens. Such stimuli are almost impossible to avoid completely in everyday life, although symptoms can improve with rigorous measures. It is sensible to try to reduce the exposure to known allergens as much as possible. In children at risk of asthma it may be particularly important to limit their exposure to potential allergic problems.

Efficacy in pollen sensitivity

There is some evidence that desensitisation is beneficial in patients with asthma who are sensitive to pollens and that repeated courses increase the improvement. Controlled studies in adults sensitive to house dust mites have shown no benefit from desensitisation. Several studies in children have suggested some benefit, but these were highly selected groups; it is unusual to find asthmatic patients with a single sensitivity. The degree of control produced by desensitisation can usually be achieved with simple, safe, inhaled drugs.

Newer techniques such as peptide immunotherapy raise the possibility of more effective and safer treatment using higher doses of modified antigen.

Drawbacks

There is little sound evidence to support desensitisation to other agents in asthmatic patients. In particular, cocktails produced from the results of skin or radioallergosorbent tests are not a valid form of treatment. Local reactions to desensitising agents are common and more generalised reactions and even death can occur. Most deaths are related to errors in the injection schedule and inadequate supervision after injections. Desensitisation should be undertaken only where appropriate facilities for resuscitation are available.

Other challenges

One area where desensitisation is appropriate is in sensitivity to insect venom that results in anaphylaxis rather than asthma. Aspirin-induced asthma may respond to careful oral desensitisation.

Combined preparations

Some fixed dose combinations are available for the treatment of asthma. Combinations of bronchodilators may be used when such treatment has been shown to be appropriate in drug and in dose. This is unusual in asthma. Combinations of short acting bronchodilators and prophylactic drug do not fit easily into most guidelines for the treatment of asthma.

Combinations of long acting inhaled bronchodilators and corticosteroids are now available and may be convenient in chronic stable asthma. It has been suggested that they may improve compliance with the prophylaxis, but this remains to be proven. Combinations potentially take away flexibility of treatment, such as doubling inhaled steroids with upper respiratory infections. Several oral combinations are available, often with small doses of theophylline, ephedrine and barbiturate. There is no indication for such preparations.

Other treatments

Many asthmatics turn to alternative therapies in the management of their asthma. Most will use these alongside conventional treatments. There have been dramatic claims for the benefit of yoga, reflexology, hypnosis, homeopathy,

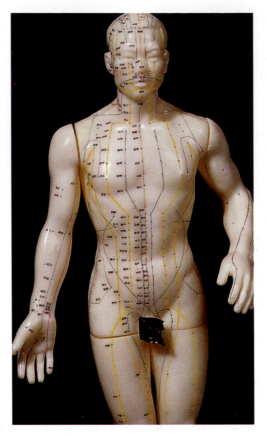

Acupuncture can be used to complement conventional therapy

Combinations of long acting β_2-agonists and steroids are available. The advantages of convenience and, possibly, compliance must be balanced against reduced flexibility

acupuncture and breathing control such as the Buteyko technique. The dangers come when these alternatives are used instead of standard treatments since few have been shown to be effective in controlled trials and none have any proven effect in prevention or treatment of severe asthma.

Relaxation

Relaxation may help to reduce the anxiety and hyperventilation that can exacerbate asthma. Such techniques may be useful in dealing with exacerbations. Patients' worries about the future course of asthma and its dangers should be explored and dealt with.

Ionisation

Ionisation of inspired air may have a small effect on lung function and may attenuate the response to exercise, but such effects are minimal and not achieved by home ionisers.

Herbal preparations

Some herbal remedies may contain useful ingredients that need investigation. Some contain conventional agents, but these are not standardised; some even contain corticosteroids and have produced the expected side-effects.

Future possibilities

There are other exciting possibilities of drugs that affect the inflammatory pathway or modulate the immunological response. Some of these are the subject of current therapeutic trials. Monoclonal antibodies against IgE may inhibit IgE synthesis, block binding or remove it from cell surfaces. Promising results have been obtained in early studies. Interleukin 5 from Th2 lymphocytes is important in attracting eosinophils to the airway and increasing responsiveness.

Drugs to reduce the production of interleukin 5, or to block its effect, are a target for development. Further back in the process is the development of uncommitted T cells to Th1 or Th2. Agents such as interleukin 12, or extracts from intracellular parasites, might drive uncommitted T cells to the Th1 pathway, reducing the inflammatory contribution from Th2 cells. T cell monoclonal antibodies are another possibility but all these modulations of the immune response will need careful safety testing.

Inhibitors of tryptase (a serine protease released from mast cells) and nitric oxide production are other areas under active investigation. It is likely that the range of such treatments available will increase over the next few years.

References

1. Results from FACET international study group. Pauwels RA, Lofdahl CG, Postma DS, Tattersfield AE, O'Byrne P, Barnes PJ, Ullman A. Effect of inhaled formoterol and budesonide on exacerbations of asthma. Formoterol and Corticosteroids Establishing Therapy (FACET) International Study Group. *N Engl J Med* 1997;**337**:1405–11.
2. Leach CL. *Respir Med* 1998;**92** suppl A: 3–8.

10   Methods of delivering drugs

Various devices and formulations have been developed to deliver drugs efficiently, minimise side-effects and simplify use. With the range of devices now available it is possible for nearly all patients to take drugs by inhalation. In some circumstances oral treatment is needed and it can be given by slow acting or sustained release preparations. Some drugs are available only by the oral route.

Metered dose inhalers

Inhalers deliver the drug directly to the airways. A metered dose inhaler (MDI) used properly deposits about 10% of the drug into the airways below the larynx. Nearly all the rest of the drug gets no further than the oropharynx and is swallowed. This swallowed portion may be absorbed from the gastrointestinal tract but drugs such as inhaled corticosteroids are largely removed by first pass metabolism in the liver. Absorption directly from the lung bypasses liver metabolism.

Patient education

An important point in the prescription of inhalation treatment is the instruction of the patient in the technique. An MDI should be shaken, then fired into the mouth shortly after the start of a slow full inspiration. At full inflation the breath should be held for 10 seconds. The technique should be checked periodically. About a quarter of patients have difficulty using a metered dose inhaler and the problems increase with age. Arthritic patients who find it hard to exert the pressure on the inhaler may be helped by a Haleraid device, which responds to squeezing, or they can be given a breath actuated or dry powder system.

CFC-free inhalers

Most current MDIs contain chlorofluorocarbon (CFC) propellants. The production, import and use of CFCs have been stopped in most developed countries because of the effect on the ozone layer. There is a temporary exemption for medical use under the Montreal Protocol, but inhalers will change from CFC use over the next few years in most countries once adequate non-CFC products become available.

Alternative propellants

The challenge has been to develop safe alternatives that are as convenient, effective and clinically equivalent. One alternative is to change to dry powder devices but this would be a tremendous educational challenge with over 400 million metered dose inhalers prescribed annually worldwide.

The process of development of alternative propellants has been more of a problem than first appreciated, particularly for inhaled steroids. Adaptations to the method of adding the drug to the propellant and to the valve and jet mechanisms have been necessary. Hydrofluoroalkanes 134 and 227 are used in the new devices and they may have some other advantages over CFCs in a more consistent particle size at low temperatures. CFC-free salbutamol and beclomethasone are now available.

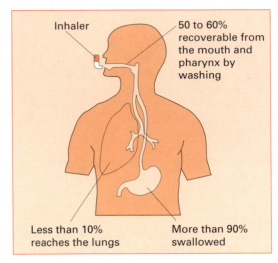

Inhalers deliver the drug direct to the airways

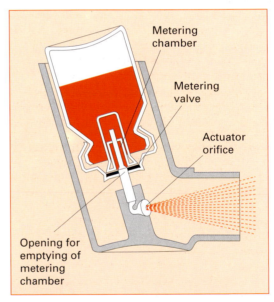

The mechanisms inside a metered dose inhaler

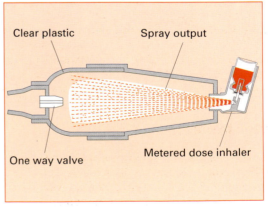

An extension tube used with a metered dose inhaler

Each new device has to be tested carefully since total and regional delivery to the lung will differ with the new devices. The beclomethasone product QVar is prescribed at half the dose of a conventional MDI because of its better lung deposition. Patients will notice differences in the speed of the aerosol cloud and taste.

The switch to CFC-free MDIs will be a great educational challenge for patients, their doctors and nurses. It should be taken as an opportunity to review patient understanding, inhaler technique and general asthma management.

Breath actuated aerosol inhalers

Breath actuated aerosol inhalers are available for most classes of drug. They are loaded by a lever (Autohaler) or by opening the cap (Easibreathe). The valve on the inhaler is actuated as the patient breathes in. The devices respond to a low inspiratory flow rate and are useful for those who have difficulty co-ordinating actuation and breathing; generally, they seem to increase lung deposition of drug. They require a propellant similar to that used in a standard inhaler.

Extension tubes

The co-ordination of firing and inspiration becomes slightly less important when a short extension tube is used. This may help if problems are minor but a larger reservoir removes the need for co-ordination of breathing and actuation. The inhaler is fixed into the chamber and the breath is taken from a one-way valve at the other end of the chamber. Inhalation should be within 30 seconds of the actuation of the inhaler.

Pharyngeal deposition is greatly reduced as the faster particles strike the walls of the chamber, not the mouth. Evaporation of propellant from the larger, slower particles produces a small-sized aerosol that penetrates further out into the lungs and deposits a greater proportion of drug beyond the larynx. This reduces the risk of oral candidiasis and dysphonia with inhaled corticosteroids and reduces potential problems with systemic absorption from the gastrointestinal tract. They should be used routinely when doses of inhaled steroid of more than 800 micrograms daily are given by metered dose inhaler.

The device is cumbersome, but this is no great disadvantage for corticosteroid treatment, which is usually given only twice a day. Chambers have proved useful as a substitute for a nebuliser in acute asthma. Output characteristics of MDIs vary and inhalers and extension tubes need to be matched appropriately. It cannot be assumed that results transfer to different combinations. The output from a chamber is affected by the electrostatic charge. This can be minimised by washing in standard household detergents.

Dry powder inhalers

Dry powder inhalers of various types are available for β-agonists, sodium cromoglycate, corticosteroids and anticholinergic agents. Because inspiratory airflow releases the fine powder many problems of co-ordination are avoided and there are none of the environmental worries of

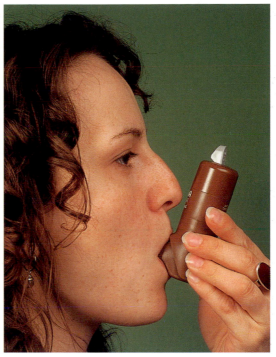

Breath-actuated inhalers are useful for patients who find it difficult to co-ordinate actuation and breathing

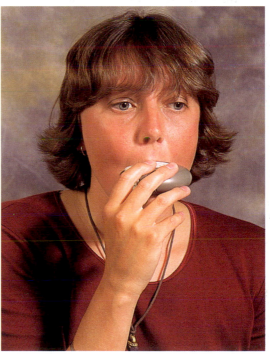

The Accuhaler has a convenient dose counter

metered dose inhalers. The dry powder makes some patients cough, however. The problems of reloading for each dose have been eased by the development of multiple dose units with up to 200 doses. Devices such as the Accuhaler and Clickhaler have a convenient dose counter that helps the patient to know when the inhaler needs renewing and provides a compliance monitor.

Dry powder devices such as the Turbohaler increase lung deposition above 20% of the dose and may allow a reduction in the prescribed dose.

Nebulisers

Nebulisers can be driven by compressed gas (jet nebuliser) or an ultrasonically vibrating crystal (ultrasonic nebuliser). They provide a way of giving inhaled drugs to those unable to use any other device – for example, the very young – or in acute attacks when inspiratory flow is limited.

Nebulisers also offer a convenient way of delivering a higher dose to the airways. Generally, about 12% of the drug leaving the chamber enters the lungs but most of the dose stays in the apparatus or is wasted in expiration. Delivery depends on the type of nebuliser chamber, the flow rate at which it is driven and the volume in the chamber. In most cases flow rates of less than 6 l/min in a jet nebuliser give too large a particle and nebulise too slowly. Some chambers have a reservoir and valve system to reduce loss to the surrounding room during expiration.

New hand-held liquid aerosol generators are in development. They act as the equivalent of hand-held nebulisers and offer a future alternative to MDIs and dry powder devices.

Tablets and syrups

Tablets and syrups are available for oral use. This route is necessary for theophyllines and leukotriene antagonists, which cannot be inhaled effectively. Very young children who are unable to inhale drugs can take the sugar-free liquid preparations. Slow release tablets are used when a prolonged action is needed, particularly for nocturnal asthma in which theophyllines have proved helpful. Various slow release mechanisms or long acting drugs have been developed to maintain even blood concentrations.

Injections and infusions

Injections are used for the treatment of acute attacks. Subcutaneous injections may be useful in emergencies when nebulisers are unavailable. Occasional patients with severe chronic asthma seem to benefit from the high levels of β-stimulant obtained with subcutaneous infusion through a portable pump. Rates may need to be adjusted depending on severity. The infusion site is changed by the patient every one to three days.

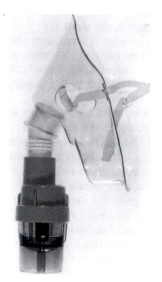

The use of nebulisers must be associated with careful instructions on use and hygiene, as well as arrangements for maintenance and support

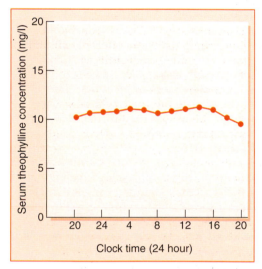

Steady theophylline concentrations in the therapeutic range can be obtained with twice daily slow release preparations (D'Alonzo D *et al*, *Am Rev Respir Dis* 1990;**142**:84–90)

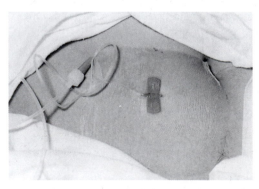

In severe cases β-agonists can be delivered by subcutaneous infusion

ASTHMA IN CHILDREN – Dipak Kanabar

11　Definition, prevalence and prevention

Defining asthma in children

Childhood asthma contains a spectrum of disorders that exhibit the clinical and pathological features as set out in the adjacent panel. Labelling a child as an asthmatic can still cause anxiety within the family and controversy among paediatricians. However, alternative diagnoses such as wheezy bronchitis or allergic airways disease probably hinder clinicians in their approach to management of asthma.

Presenting symptoms

For the majority of practising paediatricians and general practitioners, a pre-school child with recurrent wheezy episodes whose wheeze disappears following bronchodilator therapy probably justifies a clinical diagnosis of asthma (on the understanding that this term has no implications for long-term prognosis or underlying pathology).

For example, respiratory syncytial virus bronchiolitis itself causes wheezing and up to 50% of affected children will go on to develop recurrent episodic wheeze. Many children have mild wheezing during viral infections (virus associated wheeze), but their prognosis is better than children who have wheeze without a viral infection.[2] In addition, the airways of children in the first two to three years of life are small relative to lung size. Their airways and chest walls are less rigid, so during expiration they are more likely than those of older children to collapse or become obstructed by secretions or mucosal changes that are not the result of an inflammatory process like asthma.

Older children can describe symptoms of cough, wheeze, dyspnoea and chest tightness, and whether there is an improvement with bronchodilator and steroid therapy. In addition, peak flow measurements, FEV_1 by spirometry, exercise testing and recordings of diurnal variations will assist diagnosis.

Thus in paediatric practice, in the absence of an easily recognised diagnostic marker, a clinical diagnosis of asthma usually relies on a combination of history of characteristic symptoms and evidence of airway lability; in particular a reduction in symptoms after treatment with a β_2-agonist, showing reversible airflow obstruction.

Prevalence of asthma

Asthma is the most common chronic disease of childhood. One in seven children aged between 2 and 15 years in the United Kingdom has asthma symptoms requiring treatment.

Increasing prevalence

Several epidemiological studies show that the prevalence of asthma is increasing in many countries throughout the world.[3] This rise in asthma is paralleled by a rise in the prevalence of other atopic disorders such as eczema and hayfever.[4]

The International Consensus Report on the Diagnosis and Management of Asthma[1] gives the following definition. "Asthma is a chronic inflammatory disorder of the airway in which many cells play a role, in particular mast cells, eosinophils, and T lymphocytes. In susceptible individuals this inflammation causes recurrent episodes of wheezing, breathlessness, chest tightness, and cough particularly at night and or in the early morning. These symptoms are usually associated with widespread but variable airflow limitation that is at least partly reversible either spontaneously or with treatment. The inflammation also causes an associated increase in airway responsiveness to a variety of stimuli."

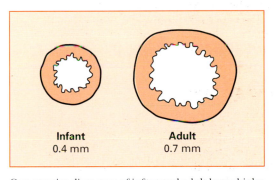

Infant	Adult
0.4 mm	0.7 mm

Comparative diameters of infant and adult bronchioles

The observation that all forms of allergic disease are increasing simultaneously suggests an increase in host susceptibility, rather than a rise in allergic sensitisation. Associations between the prevalence of asthma and small family size, affluence and BCG status (decreased asthma with BCG vaccine) are all recognised and, coupled with our understanding of the immunology of asthma, hint at the possibility of factors before birth or soon afterwards that might modify the atopic tendency of an individual.

The ISAAC study (see adjacent panel) suggested that asthma prevalence was not directly related to air pollution. Regions such as China and eastern Europe, with high levels of particulate matter and sulphur dioxide pollution, had low rates of asthma prevalence, whereas western Europe and the United States, with high levels of ozone, had an intermediate prevalence of asthma. Centres with the lowest degrees of air pollution, such as New Zealand, had a high prevalence of asthma.

Public health issues

In terms of burden of disease, childhood asthma presents a serious public health problem. More than half of all cases of asthma present before the age of 10 years and over 30% of children experience a wheezing illness during the first few years of life.[6] More absence from school is caused by asthma than any other chronic condition: 30% of asthmatic children miss more than three weeks of schooling each year. Asthma influences educational attainment even in children of above average intelligence, the extent of this adverse effect being related to severity of the disease.

Reasons for the increasing prevalence of childhood asthma

It is unlikely that that there is a single cause and effect relationship to account for the rise in prevalence of asthma and atopic disorders. However, recent immunological studies suggest that the first three years of life (including *in utero* life) are probably the most critical in terms of environmental influences on the development of the asthma phenotype. For example, there are strong links between cigarette smoking in pregnancy and narrow airways in the offspring, as well as a greater maternal versus paternal allergy risk associated with the development of asthma.

Changes such as those in housing that allow proliferation of house dust mite, the effects of outdoor and indoor pollutants such as cigarette smoke, dietary changes, low birth weight and prematurity may all account for some of the increased prevalence. However, in order to account for the increase in disease prevalence from 10% to 15% (such as has occurred in the United Kingdom since the late 1960s), the proportion of the population exposed to these hazards would need to have increased from 10% to nearly 70% suggesting that other, as yet unidentified, risk factors may be operating.

The relevance of atopy

Atopy, defined as the predisposition to raise specific IgE to common allergens, is probably the single strongest risk factor for asthma, carrying up to a 20-fold increased risk of asthma in atopic individuals compared with non-atopic individuals.

The International Study of Asthma and Allergies in Childhood (ISAAC),[5] attempted to identify further important environmental risk factors in the pathogenesis of asthma and related atopic disorders, being a population-based study spanning 56 countries with 155 centres taking part. Nearly half a million children aged 13 to 14 years completed a written questionnaire on symptoms of asthma, allergic conjunctivitis and atopic eczema; over 300 000 completed a video questionnaire. The highest prevalence of asthma symptoms was from the United Kingdom, New Zealand and Australia, with a consistently high prevalence of other atopic disorders such as eczema and hayfever

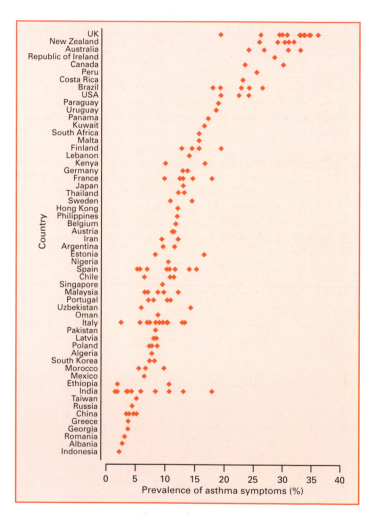

Prevalence of self-reported asthma symptoms from written questionnaires (12 month period)[5]

Lymphocytes

T lymphocytes – in particular, T-helper type 2 (Th2) lymphocytes – are also believed to be important in the pathogenesis of asthma. The fetal immune system is primarily polarised towards a Th2 response as a result of interleukin 4 and 10 (IL-4 and IL-10) production by the placenta. Furthermore, T lymphocytes isolated from cord blood of new-born babies of atopic mothers are able to respond to aeroallergens, suggesting that they may have been exposed to antigens ingested by the mother and transferred across the placenta in the last trimester of pregnancy.

During early childhood, it is believed that environmental allergens – in particular intestinal microflora – influence the immune deviation of T helper cells towards the Th1 type in non-atopic children and towards the Th2 type in atopic children. In atopic children with recurrent wheezing illness, bronchoalveolar lavage studies indicate increased mast cell and eosinophil concentrations in children as young as 3 years. Up to the age of 10, the peripheral blood mononuclear cell response to specific stimulation in children who develop atopic disease is deficient in its capacity to generate interferon gamma (IFNγ), thereby causing up-regulation of Th2 responses and an allergic phenotype. Exposure to relevant allergens in infancy or childhood may predispose to continued allergic responses later.[7]

Early exposure to infections

The "hygiene hypothesis" argues that the increase in asthma is due to a decrease in exposure to infection in early life. Frequent infections in childhood generate Th1 cytokines such as the interleukins IL-12, IL-18 and IFNγ, and these in turn inhibit the growth of Th2 cells, thus preventing development of the asthma phenotype. The hypothesis would also explain the inverse relationship between socio-economic status and asthma and allergy, with the assumption that children from higher social classes are exposed to fewer infections in early life. It may also explain why firstborn children have a higher prevalence of asthma as they would be exposed to fewer infections from siblings.

Prospects for prevention

A study designed to answer the question as to whether asthma can be avoided was carried out on the Isle of Wight in infants born to mothers with a strong family history of atopy.[8] Expectant mothers were randomised to two groups.

One group (n=58) received prophylaxis with the mothers eating a hypoallergenic diet and breast feeding, or giving a soya milk preparation to their babies. In addition, this group had reduced exposure to house dust mite by encasing childrens' mattresses and treating the house with an acaricide on four occasions. A control group (n=62) was fed conventionally by breast or on formula; no specific environmental measures were taken.

A significant decrease in the prevalence of eczema and skin prick test to aeroallergen and dietary factors was found in the prophylactic group. At the age of 4 years, the prevalence of doctor diagnosed asthma was 24.1% in the prophylactic group compared with 35.5% in the control

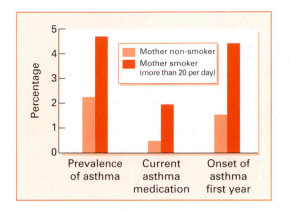

Maternal smoking and asthma in children aged 0 to 5 years, based on a 1981 NHS interview survey (n = 4331) (Dold S *et al, Arch Dis Child* 1992;**67**:1018–22)

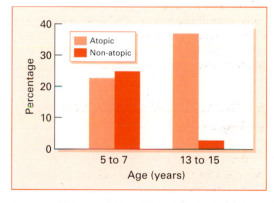

Atopy in children with bronchial hyperreactivity (Crane J *et al, J All Clin Immunol* 1989;**84**:768)

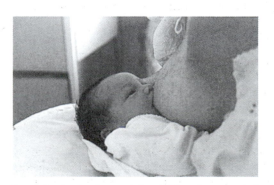

Breast feeding is advocated for children from atopic families

group. However, this difference was not significant. Other similar studies have shown equivocal results, but breast feeding is still advised in children from atopic families, or in babies identified by high cord blood IgE. Breast feeding mothers are also advised to avoid allergens to which they are sensitive.

It appears from these results that the development of asthma is a combination of genetic susceptibility and an early life exposed to allergic stimuli and pollutants that augment a Th2 immune response. Once the asthma is established, cycles of acute and chronic inflammation triggered by allergens, viruses, pollutants, diet and stress are responsible for exacerbations.

Primary preventative measures to reduce risk might therefore include allergen avoidance, cessation of smoking and attenuation of a Th2 response by vaccination. However, once asthma is established, T cells and eosinophil responses may have enhanced capacity to generate the leukotrienes IL-3, IL-4 and IL-5 and may make it more difficult to reverse an established Th2 response. In this situation, secondary prevention measures to reduce exposure to trigger factors are appropriate.

Trigger factors in asthma

During pre-school years viral infections, exercise and emotional upset are common triggers of asthma. Young children contract six to eight viral upper respiratory tract infections each year so it is not surprising that these infections are more common precipitants of asthma in children than in adults. Asthmatic children tend to have more symptoms during the winter than the summer, probably because viral respiratory infections are more common in winter and because exercise-induced asthma is more likely to develop outdoors in cold weather.

The domestic environment
Asthmatics sensitised to house dust mite for example, could reduce exposure by removal of carpets or regular hoovering, damp dusting surfaces and furniture, encasing mattresses and pillows in plastic sheets and frequently washing covers, blankets, duvets and furry toys. Reduction of humid atmospheres with dehumidifiers may be of some help. However, short- and medium-term trials of these interventions in established asthmatics have not shown benefit, but they may help in younger children at risk, or if carried out over prolonged periods.[9] Ownership of furry pets has also been shown to be related to severe asthma in adolescence, yet compliance with recommendations to remove pets is poor.

Smoking
Tobacco smoke has consistently been found to trigger exacerbation of asthma in children and families should be encouraged to stop smoking, or smoke in areas away from children and outside the house. In addition, there is a two-fold risk of developing asthma in children whose mothers smoke more than 15 cigarettes a day.

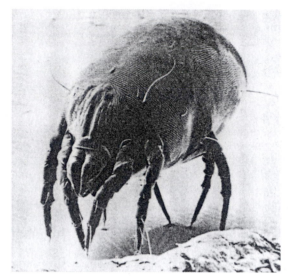
Electron micrograph of a house dust mite

Trigger factors in asthma
- Viral infections
- Dusts and pollutants including cigarette smoke
- Allergens – house dust mite, pollens, moulds, spores, animal dander and feathers, certain foods, *Alternaria* in dry arid conditions
- Exercise
- Changes in weather patterns and cold air
- Psychological factors such as stress and emotion

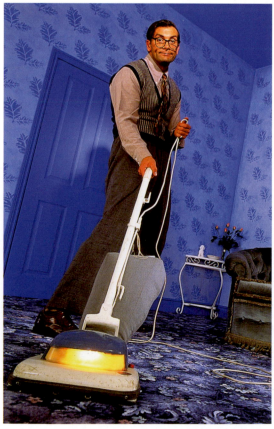
Vacuuming and other measures can make a house more bearable for children with asthma Photo: Tony Stone Images

Air pollution

Epidemiological studies have suggested that outdoor air pollution increases the severity of childhood asthma. For example, children living in polluted areas of Spain and Scandinavia have more frequent attacks of asthma than those living in unpolluted regions. So far it has not been possible to define effects of the individual components of outdoor atmospheric pollution.

Intervention

Tertiary prevention includes the provision of up-to-date guidelines to improve bronchodilation and reduce inflammation and improve quality of life.

In addition, airway remodelling may occur early in the course of disease and may then lead to irreversible loss of pulmonary function. The early administration of topical steroids may modify this development.

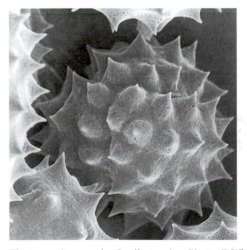

Mechanisms of mast cell and eosinophil dependent airway hyperresponsiveness[10]

Airway inflammation

Fibreoptic bronchoscopy, biopsy and bronchoalveolar lavage in the airways of asthmatic adults have shown that there is an inflammatory cellular infiltrate even when they are free of symptoms. This has led to the concept that asthma is a chronic inflammatory disorder. Eosinophils and mast cells are the important effector cells, the inflammatory process being modulated by T lymphocytes and macrophages and amplified by neural mechanisms.

Indirect evidence of an inflammatory process in the airways of young children has come from measurement of markers of inflammation in the blood and bronchoalveolar lavage, but few histological studies are available in children. However, the airways of children who have died of their asthma have shown an intense inflammatory response. We do not know how or when the inflammatory process starts, at what stage it becomes irreversible, or even whether the same type of inflammatory response occurs in all young wheezy children.

No component of the inflammatory process can be used as a diagnostic test for childhood asthma or as a reliable way to assess response to treatment. Diagnosis and the choice of treatment still depend on clinical judgement based on the nature, frequency and severity of symptoms combined with physiological assessment of airway function.

Electron micrograph of pollen grains Photo: R Whitenstall

References

1. International Consensus Report on the Diagnosis and Management of Asthma. *Clin Exper Allergy* 1992;**22** suppl 1.

2. Godden *et al.* Outcome of wheeze in childhood. *Am J Respir Crit Care Med* 1994;**149**:106–112.

3. Russell G, Helms PJ. Trends in occurrence of asthma among children and young adults. *BMJ* 1997;**315**:1014–15.

4. Aberg N, Hesselmar B, Aberg B, Eriksson B. Increase of asthma, allergic rhinitis and eczema in Swedish schoolchildren between 1979 and 1991. *Clin Exp Allergy* 1995;**25**:815–19.

5. ISAAC Steering Committee. *Lancet* 1998;**351**:1225–31.

6. Glezen WP. Epidemiological patterns of acute lower respiratory tract disease of children in a paediatric group practice. *J Paediatr* 1971;**78**:397–406.

7. Holt PG, Clough JB, Holt BJ *et al.* Genetic "risk" for atopy is associated with delayed postnatal maturation of T cell competence. *Clin Exp Allergy* 1992;**22**:1093–9.

8. Hide DW, Matthews S, Tariq S, Arshad SH. Allergen avoidance in infancy and allergy at 4 years of age. *Allergy* 1996;**51**:89–93.

9. Custovic A, Simpson A, Chapman MD, Woodcock A. Allergen avoidance in the treatment of asthma and atopic disorders. *Thorax* 1998;**53**:63–72.

10. Drazen JM, Arm JP, Austen KF. Sorting Out the Cytokines of Asthma. *J Exp Med* 1996;**183**:1–5.

12   Patterns of illness and diagnosis

Wheezing in infancy

As discussed in chapter 11, young children up to the age of 3 years are particularly prone to wheezing illnesses.

Martinez (see adjacent panel) was able to differentiate early transient wheezers from persistent wheezers by analysis of risk factors and lung function tests. The transient wheezers had smaller airways and their mothers smoked, whereas the persistent wheezers had a more classical atopic history with a positive family history of maternal asthma, raised serum IgE and positive skin prick tests.

Respiratory tract infections

Many babies have repeated episodes of wheezing associated with viral respiratory tract infections. The mechanism by which this happens is still not fully understood but genetic constitution and environmental influences in early life may predispose to wheeze by causing changes in airway calibre or in lung function. For example, wheezy lower respiratory illnesses are more common among boys, among infants or parents who smoke and among babies born prematurely who have needed prolonged positive pressure ventilation. Thus pre-existing factors other than asthma that cause narrowing of the airways account for more than a half of the wheezing developed by infants.

Bronchiolitis

About 1% of infants are admitted to hospital with acute viral bronchiolitis. Recurrent cough and wheezing commonly follow, but in most cases stop before school age. About 40% of babies with atopic eczema also develop recurrent wheezing and there is a strong association between a family history of atopic disease and wheezing in early childhood. According to the data from Martinez 14% of children had persistent wheezing from infancy to the age of 6 years (persistent wheezers); this group also had the highest proportion of viral respiratory disease in the first year of life suggesting that some viral infections may facilitate the development of asthma as well as being responsible for its prevention.

Asthma progression from childhood to adolescence

The outcome of early onset wheeze is still controversial. Children seen in referral centres have poorer outcomes than those followed up in longitudinal studies of general populations, probably as a result of more severe asthma being referred to hospital.

Predictability

The data from Martinez would suggest that early onset asthma is associated with poor outcome in terms of lung function and persistent bronchial hyper-responsiveness. Another study in infants aged 1 month showed that those who were more responsive to histamine challenge were more likely to have asthma diagnosed at the age of 6 years,[2] and other studies have shown a clear

A prospective study by Martinez[1] looked at over 1200 children born in Tucson, Arizona. In 826 children, at 6 years of age, 51% had never wheezed. In the others, three patterns were identified, 20% of children who wheezed early on with respiratory tract infections had no wheezing by the age of 6 years (early transient group); 15% had no wheezing at the age of 3 years but had wheezing at the age of 6 years (late onset group); and 14% had wheezing before the age of 3 years and at the age of 6 years (persistent wheezers)

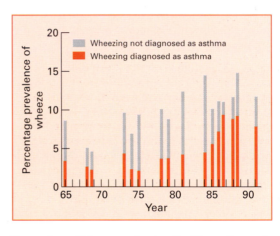

Comparison of 16 surveys showing the 12 month prevalence of wheezing diagnosed or not diagnosed as asthma in children (1965–91) (Anderson HR, *Paed Resp Med* 1993;**1**:6–10)

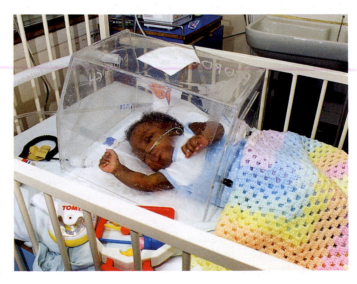

About 1% of infants will be admitted to hospital with acute viral bronchiolitis

relationship between degree of airway hyper-responsiveness to histamine challenge and persistence of asthma.[3]

However, data from Jenkins, who reviewed a group of patients aged 29 to 32 years who had previously been studied at the age of 7 years by questionnaire and spirometry, suggested that of those who had reported asthma at age 7, 26% were still symptomatic as adults.[4] Other childhood risk factors that predicted asthma in adult life included being female, a family history of asthma and more severe asthma (especially if it developed after the age of 2 and was associated with reduced expiratory flow rate).

A population study in New Zealand reported that as children grow older bronchial hyper-reactivity decreases. Judged by the response to inhaled histamine, the number of children with hyper-responsive airways halved between the ages of 6 and 12. In contrast the total number of children with atopy doubled. Of those between the ages of 5 and 7 who had evidence of bronchial reactivity about 50% were atopic; of the children aged 13 with bronchial hyper-responsiveness over 90% were atopic.

Results of studies

These results support the clinical observations that non-specific factors, notably viral infections and exercise, are important triggers of asthma during pre-school years and allergic triggers assume greater importance as children grow older. Other similar longitudinal studies suggest that children with mild disease usually outgrow their asthma as a result of the increase in airway size with growth and the apparent spontaneous decline in airway responsiveness with age. However, females and those with more severe disease, greater airway hyper-responsiveness and an atopic history have persistent disease.

Teenagers with asthma

The prevalence of asthma by self report among teenagers aged 13 to 14 years was as high as 30% in the United Kingdom. In the ISAAC study, the prevalence of doctor diagnosed asthma in 12 to 14 year olds in the United Kingdom was 21%, suggesting that asthma is under-diagnosed in this age group. In addition, between 1990 and 1992, mortality in 10 to 14 year olds was three times the mortality of 5 to 9 year olds and in teenagers 15 to 19 years of age was six times the rate in 5 to 9 year olds, suggesting that treatment or compliance was suboptimal.[5]

Asthmatic teenagers are coping with a period of intense emotional and psychological change and this can have a significant impact on quality of life. They also have concerns about body image, peer acceptance, physical capabilities in terms of exercise and activity, and the physiological delay of puberty caused by their asthma, all of which can complicate their asthma treatment goals. In addition, because of a need to emphasise their own identity, they may become isolated and may suffer from anxiety and depression, especially if they are excluded from participation in the decision making process regarding their condition. They may also participate in risky behaviour such as cigarette smoking and non-compliance with treatment, which may account for their increased morbidity and mortality.

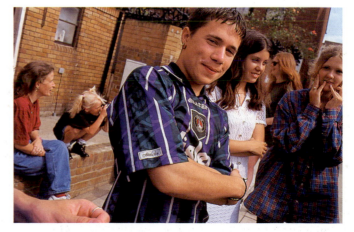

Asthma is often under-diagnosed in younger teenagers

Sympathetic consultation

Paediatricians need to recognise the needs of these vulnerable teenagers by spending more time listening to them, helping them making choices of treatment and negotiating a plan of action that allows for compromise on both sides. Holding separate young person clinics and being prepared to discuss wider issues than asthma may go some way to improve understanding and compliance. The goals of treatment are psychological well being, allowing full physical activity and minimal effects on the underlying developmental progression from childhood to adulthood.

Diagnosis of asthma

The diagnosis of asthma is made following an appropriate clinical history and examination, testing for reversibility of bronchoconstriction and assessing a response to therapy. Demonstrating airway reversibility or a short-term trial with anti-asthma therapy may be useful diagnostic markers especially in those children with episodic symptoms.

Presentation

In school-age children there is little difficulty in recognising asthma, especially when one asks specifically about cough, wheeze, shortness of breath and exercise-induced symptoms. Pre-school children sometimes present with cough alone. The other characteristics that suggest asthma are episodic cough or wheeze, and symptoms worsening at night, after exercise, after exposure to allergens or with viral respiratory tract infections. Asthmatic babies sometimes have attacks of breathlessness without obvious wheezing.

Hypersecretory asthma

Some asthmatic children produce large amounts of bronchial secretions. This is called hypersecretory asthma. Increased production of mucus is associated with a productive cough, airway plugging and areas of collapse on the chest radiograph. These children may be misdiagnosed as having recurrent lower respiratory tract infection.

The vast majority of wheezing in infancy is due to accumulation of secretions in the airway in response to bronchial inflammation. However, certain features suggest that the cough or wheezing may be caused by factors other than asthma. These include onset in the new-born period, chronic diarrhoea or failure to thrive, recurrent infections, choking or difficulty with swallowing, mediastinal or focal abnormalities on the chest radiograph and the presence of cardiovascular abnormalities.

Lung function tests

When possible the diagnosis should be confirmed by lung function testing. This can be done at any age, but in infants and very young children the facilities are available only in specialised centres. From the age of 4 years some children can use a peak flow meter and the peak flow reading can be compared with a range of values related to the child's height. A normal peak flow reading at one examination does not exclude asthma; several recordings made at home may be more valuable. Occasionally an exercise test or therapeutic trial is necessary to confirm the diagnosis. Measurement of total IgE concentration will ascertain only whether the child is atopic. A chest radiograph is more useful to look for other causes of wheezing than to diagnose asthma.

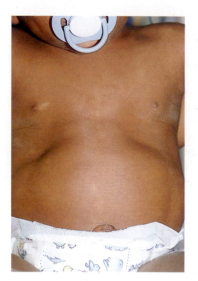

Chest deformity like this is an indication to treat with inhaled steroids

---

Other causes of noisy breathing in children
- Bronchiolitis
- Inhalation, foreign body, milk
- Gastro-oesophageal reflux
- Cystic fibrosis
- Tuberculosis
- Bronchomalacia
- Tracheal or bronchial stenosis
- Vascular rings
- Mediastinal masses

Labelling

Making a diagnosis of asthma carries with it a certain stigma, for no parent likes to be told their child may have a chronic illness with the possibility of recurrent exacerbations. However, with appropriate explanation and reassurance, parental anxiety is more likely to be reduced and compliance with therapy increased.

Assessment of severity

Ideally, the management of asthma should include serial measurement of markers of disease activity, but as yet there are none that can be applied to the clinical care of asthmatic children. Evaluation of severity and response to treatment has therefore to be made by clinical assessment complemented when possible by measurements of peak flow and lung function. A sound approach is to classify the asthma as mild, moderate, or severe; to base the initial treatment regimen on this assessment and then decide at regular reviews whether there is scope to modify medication.

Mild asthma

For asthma to be categorised as mild, symptomatic episodes should occur less frequently than once a month. Symptoms do not interfere with daytime activity or sleep. There is a good response to bronchodilator treatment; lung function returns to normal between attacks.

Moderate asthma

Children with moderate asthma have some symptoms several days a week and have attacks of asthma more than once a month but less than once a week. There is no chest deformity and growth is unaffected. Attacks may be triggered by viral infection, allergens, exercise, cigarette smoke, climatic changes and emotional upset.

Severe asthma

The third category, severe asthma, is the least common. Children have troublesome symptoms on most days, wake frequently with asthma at night, miss school and are unable to participate fully in school or outdoor activities. They may be retarded in growth and have chest deformities.

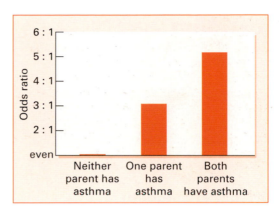

Odds ratios for asthma in children (Weitzman M *et al*, *Paediatrics* 1990;**85**:505–11)

Some children do not fit any of these categories. Seasonal asthma caused by allergy to grass pollen generally affects older children. A few children have sudden very severe attacks of asthma, which result in admission to hospital and may be life threatening, separated by long periods without symptoms during which their lung function returns to normal. This latter group is very difficult to treat.

References

1. Martinez FD, Wright AL, Taussig LM, *et al*. Asthma and wheezing in the first six years of life. The Group Health Medical Associates. *NEJM*, 1995;**332**:133–8.
2. Palmer LJ, Gibbon NA, Rye PJ *et al*. Airway responsiveness (AR) at 1 month of age predicts lung function and atopic and respiratory illness at 6 years of age. *Austr NZ J Med* 1995;**25**:412.
3. Gerritsen J, Koeter GH, Postma *et al*. Airway responsiveness in childhood as a predictor of the outcome of asthma in adulthood. *Am Rev Respir Dis* 1991;**143**:1468–9.
4. Jenkins MA, Hopper JL, Bowes G *et al*. Factors in childhood as predictors of asthma in adult life. *BMJ* 1994;**309**:90–93.
5. Office of Population, Censuses and Surveys. *Mortality Statistics 1990–1992*, **25–27**. London:HMSO.

13   Treatment

The aims of treatment are shown in the adjacent panel. They can be achieved by prompt diagnosis, identification of trigger factors, evaluation of severity, establishment of a partnership of management with the asthmatic child and the family, and regular review.

Partnership in management

Self management plans allow a partnership to be established between the doctor, the child and the family. The aim of the plan is to allow families to become more confident about the day-to-day management of asthma, to cope with exacerbations and to prevent hospital admission with early intervention, and thereby ultimately to reduce health costs. The goals of the partnership are listed below.

In young children, plans are more likely to be based on the child's symptoms than on objective assessments such as peak flow measurements. In older children, peak flow assessments are useful, especially for those who are poor perceivers of symptoms.

Other sources of information
Respiratory nurses working in asthma clinics, schools and general practice play a pivotal role in establishing this partnership, as well as keeping regular personal contact, reassuring and encouraging children and their families. In addition, there is a wealth of information available from organisations such as the National Asthma Campaign.

Changing the environment

As mentioned in chapter 11, the avoidance of cigarette smoking is especially important during pregnancy. Families with asthmatic children should be discouraged from acquiring pets. With a pet already present, the pet allergy has to be established with a good history of exacerbation following contact (as well as skin prick tests or specific IgE levels) before removal is advised. It might take several months before the animal dander completely disappears.

House dust mite
House dust mite sensitivity is the most common allergy in asthmatic children. At high altitudes where concentrations of house dust mite and other inhaled antigens are low, symptoms, bronchial reactivity and the need for medication are considerably reduced. However, only considerable environmental changes to reduce house dust mite have been shown to be effective in improving asthma.

The aims of treatment should be:
- To abolish symptoms and allow children to lead a full and active life at home and at school
- To restore normal lung function and reduce variations in peak flow
- To minimise the requirement for bronchodilator therapy
- To enable normal growth and development and avoid adverse effects of medication

The outcomes of successful self management are:
- Absence of or minimal cough, shortness of breath and wheeze, including nocturnal symptoms
- Minimal or infrequent exacerbations
- Minimal need for bronchodilator therapy
- No limitation of activity, especially exercise and games
- Restoration of normal lung function and reduced variations in peak flow
- Minimal or no adverse effects from the medication

Partnership comprises:
- An understanding of asthma and goals of treatment
- Monitoring of symptoms
- Use of a peak flow meter when appropriate
- An agreed plan of action of what to do when the child's asthma improves, gets worse, or there is an acute attack
- Clear written instructions

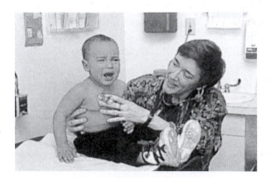

Nurses in clinics, schools and general practice help to maintain partnership in the management of childhood asthma Photo: Science Picture Library

14   Drug treatment

The BTS guidelines on asthma management (1997) propose a stepwise and algorithmic approach to drug management in paediatric asthma. There are some important points to remember when following the guidelines.

Children should start at the step most appropriate to the severity of presentation of asthma and then move up or down the steps until a minimal effective dose of inhaled steroid is achieved to control symptoms.

Before stepping up at any stage of treatment, ensure that compliance is good, that an appropriate inhaler device is given and that the inhaler technique is good. Exclude other possible diagnoses such as gastro-oesophageal reflux, bronchiolitis, foreign body inhalation and cystic fibrosis.

Rescue intervention
A rescue course of prednisolone at any step of 1 to 2 mg/kg/day is allowed for acute exacerbations for three to five days without the requirement for dose tapering. Also, during exacerbations, children are often advised to double the dose of inhaled steroid for up to four weeks until they have shown clinical improvement, following which the child can then return to the original dose. A bronchodilator can also be used more frequently after such exacerbations.

Review
Children should be reviewed every three to six months and if stable, advised to reduce the dose of inhaled steroid by 25 to 50% until a minimum effective dose is achieved.

Older children
Children older than 5 years are generally believed to require a similar approach to management as that for adults.

Bronchodilators

Children with mild episodic asthma need only intermittent treatment with bronchodilator drugs, which should be given whenever possible by inhalation (step 1 of the BTS guidelines). Those with more severe asthma who are taking a prophylactic agent should always have a fast-acting bronchodilator readily available. The selective β_2-adrenergic agonists (for example, salbutamol and terbutaline) are the best and safest bronchodilators.

Asthma in childhood is often triggered by viral respiratory tract infections and exercise. It may be necessary to take a bronchodilator regularly during and for a week or two after, a cold. If the bronchodilator has to be continued for longer, treatment with a prophylactic agent should be considered. A single dose of an inhaled β_2-adrenergic bronchodilator taken 15 to 20 minutes before a games period at school helps to prevent exercise-induced wheezing.

Nebulisers
In wheezy infants β_2-adrenergic bronchodilators inhaled through a nebuliser can be ineffective and may sometimes be associated with worsening of intrathoracic airway function: the poor response may be related to the small dose of drug reaching the airways. One study of a spacer

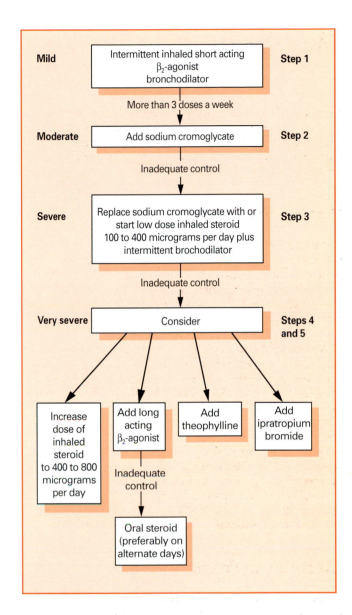

Mild	Intermittent inhaled short acting β_2-agonist bronchodilator	Step 1

More than 3 doses a week

Moderate	Add sodium cromoglycate	Step 2

Inadequate control

Severe	Replace sodium cromoglycate with or start low dose inhaled steroid 100 to 400 micrograms per day plus intermittent brochodilator	Step 3

Inadequate control

Very severe	Consider	Steps 4 and 5

Increase dose of inhaled steroid to 400 to 800 micrograms per day — Add long acting β_2-agonist — Add theophylline — Add ipratropium bromide

Inadequate control

Oral steroid (preferably on alternate days)

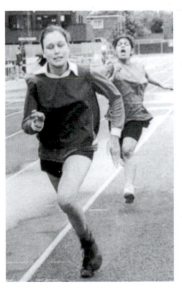

A single dose of an inhaled β_2-adrenergic bronchodilator can help to prevent exercise-induced wheezing Photo: Ulrike Preuss

device specifically designed for use in babies showed consistent improvement in lung function after salbutamol. In young children the anticholinergic agent ipratropium bromide may also be beneficial, given either through a nebuliser or a spacer device with a face mask.

Long acting β_2-agonists

Long acting β_2-agonists are available for paediatric usage at step 3 of the BTS guidelines. In the United Kingdom, salmeterol is currently licensed for use in children from the age of 4 years and eformoterol in children over the age of 12 years. They increase airway calibre for at least 12 hours and prevent exercise-induced symptoms for up to nine hours. Their safety profile is similar to that of short acting β_2-agonists. Although symptoms improve when these agents are given alone, their use is more appropriate when given in conjunction with regular anti-inflammatory therapy.

Prophylactic agents

The biggest advance in asthma therapy came with the development of topically active inhaled corticosteroids. Non-steroidal prophylactic agents include sodium cromoglycate, nedocromil sodium and leukotriene antagonists.

Indications

Lung function between attacks can be assessed by spirometric measurements of FEV_1 and forced vital capacity. More subtle abnormalities can be detected by forced expiratory flow volume curves or by measurement of lung volumes in a respiratory function laboratory.

A single measurement of peak expiratory flow rate (PEFR) may be misleading, but recordings made at home in the morning and afternoon or evening over a week or two may show variations in PEFR that indicate airway instability and the need for prophylactic medication. Once started, regular treatment with a prophylactic agent is likely to be needed for years rather than months and should be withdrawn only when there has been little need for bronchodilator treatment for at least three months. Close supervision is necessary during withdrawal of a prophylactic drug.

Leukotriene receptor antagonists

Leukotrienes are a recognised mediator of asthma as they cause bronchoconstriction, mucus secretion and increased vascular permeability promoting eosinophil migration into airways mucosa. The role of leukotriene receptor antagonists in paediatric asthma is currently being evaluated. Recent studies in children aged 6 to 14 have shown an improvement in exercise-induced bronchospasm and an improvement in FEV_1.[1, 2] Although not included in the 1997 BTS guidelines, they should possibly be considered at step 3 in combination with inhaled corticosteroids. Montelukast is licensed in the United Kingdom for children over 6 years and zafirlukast in those over 12 years of age.

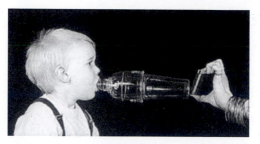
Small children can use a large volume spacer with assistance

Long-acting β_2-agonists are particularly useful in the following situations:

- When considering increasing the dose of inhaled corticosteroid therapy, one can instead use a long acting β_2-agonist together with the original lower dose of inhaled steroid
- When there are persistent nocturnal and troublesome exercise-induced symptoms

---

The following signs indicate that regular prophylactic medication should be given:

- Frequent symptoms and the need to take a bronchodilator several days a week
- Frequent nocturnal cough and wheezing even when asthma is not troublesome during the day
- At least one asthma attack a month
- Failure of lung function to return to normal between attacks

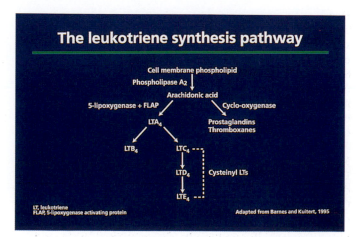
The leukotriene synthesis pathway

Sodium cromoglycate

Despite its prolonged use in childhood and adult asthma, the exact mode of action of sodium cromoglycate remains unknown. The BTS guidelines recommend it as a preventive agent for children with moderate asthma (step 2) as an alternative to low-dose inhaled steroid therapy. The metered dose aerosol is as effective as the powder in children who are able to use it properly and is slightly less likely to cause coughing after inhalation.

Nebulised cromoglycate improves asthma in pre-school children although it does not reduce hospital admission rates or severe wheezing provoked by viral respiratory infections. The apparent reduction in efficacy when cromoglycate is given by nebuliser to very young children, especially those under 1 year of age, may be because at this age only a small amount of the drug reaches the airways.

Compliance
Sodium cromoglycate is completely safe with virtually no side-effects even when taken regularly for years, which is a strong argument for using it when possible. Unfortunately its taste and the requirement for it to be taken three or four times a day make non-compliance a common reason for failure of treatment.

Evaluation
Sodium cromoglycate is unlikely to control symptoms in children with severe asthma. The response to cromoglycate should be carefully evaluated four to six weeks after starting treatment and it is important to decide whether optimal control of asthma has been achieved or merely some improvement in symptoms. If the asthma is still interfering with the child's daily activity, if the peak flow is unstable, or if the child still requires frequent relief medication, cromoglycate should be replaced by a low dose of an inhaled steroid (step 2).

Inhaled steroids

Corticosteroids are the most potent anti-inflammatory agents available for treating asthma and they have the greatest diversity of action.

Dosage
The starting dose depends on the clinical assessment of severity but in older children with frequent symptoms the usual practice is to start with a relatively high dose (400 to 800 micrograms per day of budesonide or beclomethasone, or 250 to 500 micrograms per day of fluticasone) and reducing the dose in a stepwise fashion to the minimum effective dose required to prevent symptoms (stepping down).

Methods of delivery
Inhaled steroids given by pressurised aerosol (MDI) or by dry powder inhaler are effective in older children. Combining an inhaled steroid with cromoglycate does not confer additional benefit. In recent years inhaled steroids have been used increasingly to treat asthma in pre-school children. When an inhaled steroid is given to a pre-school child with frequent or severe asthma through a large

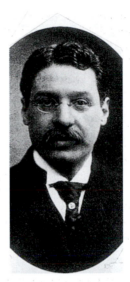

In 1900, Soloman Solis-Cohen reported the beneficial effects of oral dried bovine adrenal extract in 12 patients with asthma. This was probably the first recorded usage of steroids in asthma

---

Indications for prescribing inhaled steroids to children are:
- As first-line prophylactic therapy (BTS guidelines step 2)
- When moderate asthma, recurrent acute attacks, daily wheeze and shortness of breath are not adequately controlled by cromoglycate
- When asthma is more severe (BTS guidelines steps 3 or 4) particularly in children with chest deformity

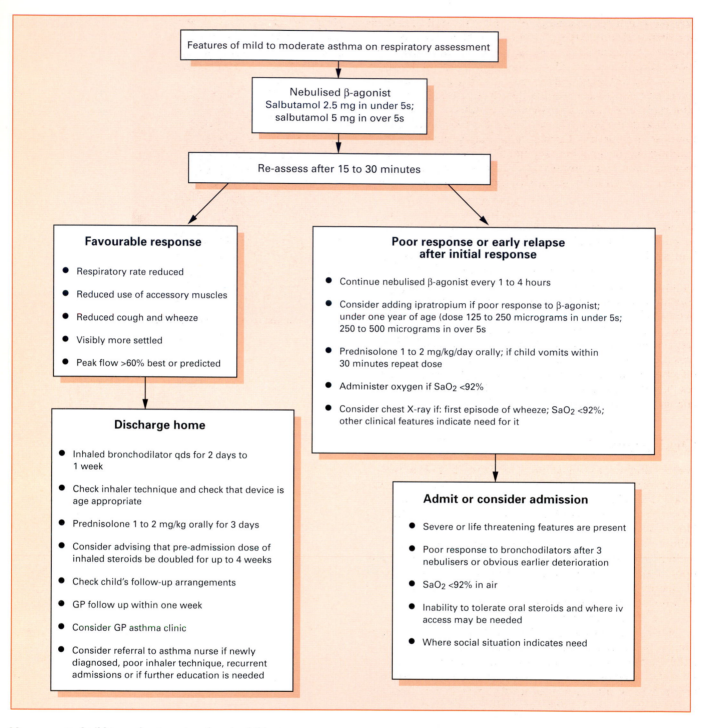

Features of mild to moderate asthma on respiratory assessment

Nebulised β-agonist
Salbutamol 2.5 mg in under 5s;
salbutamol 5 mg in over 5s

Re-assess after 15 to 30 minutes

Favourable response

- Respiratory rate reduced
- Reduced use of accessory muscles
- Reduced cough and wheeze
- Visibly more settled
- Peak flow >60% best or predicted

Discharge home

- Inhaled bronchodilator qds for 2 days to 1 week
- Check inhaler technique and check that device is age appropriate
- Prednisolone 1 to 2 mg/kg orally for 3 days
- Consider advising that pre-admission dose of inhaled steroids be doubled for up to 4 weeks
- Check child's follow-up arrangements
- GP follow up within one week
- Consider GP asthma clinic
- Consider referral to asthma nurse if newly diagnosed, poor inhaler technique, recurrent admissions or if further education is needed

Poor response or early relapse after initial response

- Continue nebulised β-agonist every 1 to 4 hours
- Consider adding ipratropium if poor response to β-agonist; under one year of age (dose 125 to 250 micrograms in under 5s; 250 to 500 micrograms in over 5s
- Prednisolone 1 to 2 mg/kg/day orally; if child vomits within 30 minutes repeat dose
- Administer oxygen if SaO$_2$ <92%
- Consider chest X-ray if: first episode of wheeze; SaO$_2$ <92%; other clinical features indicate need for it

Admit or consider admission

- Severe or life threatening features are present
- Poor response to bronchodilators after 3 nebulisers or obvious earlier deterioration
- SaO$_2$ <92% in air
- Inability to tolerate oral steroids and where iv access may be needed
- Where social situation indicates need

Management of mild to moderate acute asthma in children

volume spacer with a one-way valve and a face mask, it is as effective as in older children; this seems to be the best delivery system for the very young.

Trials of steroids given by nebuliser to young children in conventional doses (200 to 400 micrograms per day) have given disappointing results. This is almost certainly because the amount of drug delivered in a suspension from a nebuliser to a freely breathing infant or young child is small. Over three-quarters of the inhaled steroid remains in the nebuliser and fewer than 20% of the nebulised droplets containing drug are less than 5 microns in diameter. To overcome this problem it is necessary to use large starting doses; regimes of nebulised budesonide up to 1000 micrograms per day have shown a therapeutic effect in infants with severe asthma.

Adverse effects
Understandably there is a reluctance to give inhaled steroids to young children because of concern about

possible side-effects. Local side-effects such as oral candidiasis and dysphonia are rare in childhood, probably because powder inhalers and spacer devices are used. Inhaled steroids have a dose dependent effect on the adrenal glands by which they reduce resting cortisol output. It is difficult to separate the effects of asthma versus inhaled corticosteroids on children's growth, as both can adversely affect it.

Likewise, if children whose asthma is well controlled on low-dose steroids are placed on high-dose steroids, growth stunting may occur, whereas children with severe asthma may not experience any adverse effects, but instead may enjoy a good period of growth as a result of better control.

Growth

When the evidence for the effects of inhaled corticosteroids on childhood growth is examined, beclomethasone and budesonide at dosages used at step 3 or above of the BTS guidelines affect childhood growth as assessed by knemometry (leg length below the knee) and as assessed by conventional stadiometry, however, final height has not been shown to be adversely affected.[3] There is some suggestion that fluticasone may have an advantage in this respect with fewer systemic effects because of its high first pass metabolism. The exact mechanism of adverse growth effect by inhaled steroids is unknown, but believed to be the result of decreased bone turnover, rather than that due to changes in growth hormone or IGF1 levels.

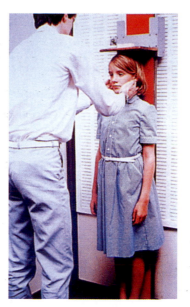

Measurement of growth in children by stadiometry

Oral agents

When a drug has to be taken regularly there are obvious advantages if it can be taken by mouth and only once or twice a day. The leukotriene antagonists have been discussed above. Slow release theophyllines in doses titrated to give blood concentrations of 10 to 20 mg/l will control asthma in children with frequent symptoms but they are relatively ineffective in preventing the wheezing that accompanies viral upper respiratory tract infections. The variable clearance rate of theophylline in children means that it is difficult to predict the dose of the drug that will give therapeutic blood concentrations in an individual child.

Side-effects (notably gastrointestinal upsets and behaviour disturbances) are common particularly in pre-school children. Because of problems with giving the drug and its side-effects, the use of theophyllines has been restricted to children whose asthma is uncontrolled despite treatment with inhaled steroids (BTS guidelines steps 4 and 5).

Inhaler devices

Whenever possible, asthma treatment should be given to children by inhalation; the most common reasons for failure of inhalation treatment are inappropriate selection or incorrect use of the inhaler. Children become fully aware of their own breathing and recognise the difference between inspiration and expiration by about the age of 3 years; until then they need inhalation devices that require only tidal breathing.

Inspiratory flow rates are slower and the airways narrower in children. Both these factors influence the dose inhaled and the site of deposition of the drug. The choice of inhaler will depend on the child's age and preference for a particular device.

Inhaler devices for children

Age	1 to 2 years	3 to 5 years	5 years or older
MDI with large volume spacer and mask	1st choice	2nd choice	–
MDI with large volume spacer	2nd choice	1st choice	2nd choice
Dry powder inhaler	Inappropriate	Occasionally useful	1st choice

Aerosols and powders

Most children under the age of 10 years are unable to achieve the co-ordination needed to use an unmodified MDI. Less than half of the children who use them obtain benefit from these devices because of poor inhalation technique. Breath actuated aerosol inhalers (Autohalers) are easier to use but a child tends to close the glottis when the breath actuated valve opens. The number that are able to use these inhalers declines rapidly under the age of 7 years.

Dry powder inhalers

Breath actuated dry powder inhalers are either single dose (Spinhaler, Rotahaler) or multiple dose (Accuhaler, Turbohaler). The age at which breath actuated powder inhalers can be used depends on the optimal inspiratory flow rate: for example the Rotahaler requires an inspiratory rate of at least 90 l/minute whereas the Turbohaler needs an inspiration of about 30 l/minute. The latter can therefore be used in children over the age of 4 to 5 years with proper training. In addition, twice as much drug can be deposited in the lungs with a Turbohaler than with the same drug given via an MDI (without a spacer).

Spacers and nebulisers

A spacer device reduces the velocity of the particles before they reach the mouth and allows more of the propellant to evaporate so that the inhaled particles become smaller and penetrate further into the lungs. Recent developments include that of a metal spacer device, which has no electrostatic charge, no dead space and may allow better lung deposition. After activation of the drug canister, the aerosol can be inhaled by taking a few breaths sufficient to open and close the valve attached to the mouthpiece. Children can use large volume spacers in this way from the age of 2 years.

Children under 2 years can be given inhalers with a large volume spacer and mask with the spacer held at 45° to keep the valve open. The infant can then inhale the medication during normal tidal respiration. During acute attacks, infants and young children may not tolerate a face mask, in which case only nebulised treatment is appropriate. Some families report that their children cannot tolerate a face mask, but a large cup or drink carton can be used in place of a spacer.

Nebulisers

Nebulisers are expensive, time consuming and inconvenient. They are often used incorrectly at home. A compressor and jet nebuliser suitable for giving asthma medication should have a driving gas flow rate of 8 to 10 l/minute and a volume fill of 4 ml; this is particularly important when giving a suspension such as an inhaled

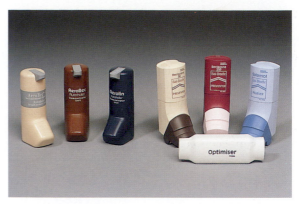
Breath actuated devices

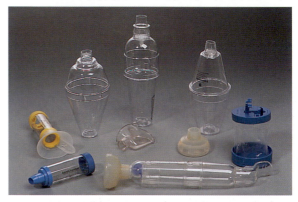
A range of spacer devices

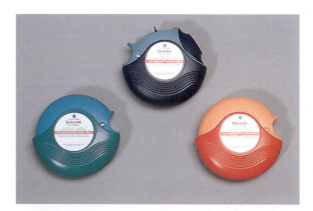
Accuhaler device

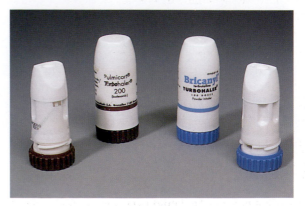
Turbohaler device

steroid. It is not justified to assume that the equivalent dose for older children is appropriate for a younger age group because inhalation technique, tidal volume breathing and the anatomy of the upper airway are different.

Despite these reservations, there is an important place for the judicious use of nebulisers in the treatment of young asthmatic children at home. A double-blind placebo-controlled study of 36 children with poorly controlled asthma, showed a significant improvement in their asthma and reduction of oral corticosteroid intake.[4]

Choice of device

Patient preference is of major importance in the choice of device. Most patients are unable to use MDIs correctly and even with good technique only 10 to 15% of the dose is delivered to the lungs.

Spacer devices will reduce co-ordination problems and improve lung deposition. Children on regular prophylactic inhaled steroids are advised to use a spacer at all times. Even when a spacer device is used, correct positioning of the device, inhalation of the drug within 10 to 20 seconds, single dose actuations and regular rinse and drip-dry of the spacer devices are important take-home instructions.

Dry powder inhalers may also vary in their lung deposition; up to 30% of a drug may reach the lungs with a good technique. The main determining factor for their use is variations in the inspiratory flow rate.

The table earlier in this chapter is a useful guide to appropriate choice of device.

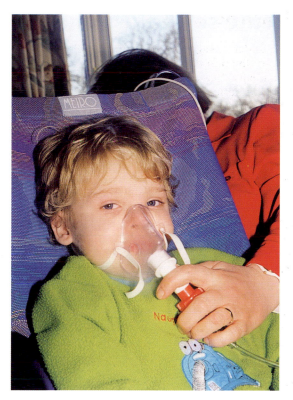

Nebulisers need to be used correctly in a domestic environment

The future

There have been some major advances in our understanding of the pathogenesis of childhood asthma. We now need to identify more precisely the factors that can prevent the onset of disease and modify disease progression.

Genetic markers should enable the identification of children at risk and allow more specific pharmacological therapies in individual cases. Immunomodulation and modification of fetal and early life environmental factors are on the horizon, but in the meantime we need to improve our and our patients' understanding of the disease, improve compliance and develop simple and better tolerated therapies with fewer systemic side-effects.

References

1. Kemp JP, Dockhorn RJ, Shapiro GC et al. Montelukast once daily inhibits exercise-induced bronchoconstriction in 6- to 14-year-old children with asthma. *Journal of Paediatrics* 1998;**133**:424–8.
2. Knor B, Matz J, Bernstein JA et al. Montelukast for chronic asthma in 6- to 14-year-old children. A randomised, double-blind trial. *JAMA* 1998;**279**:1181–6.
3. Allen DB, Mullen ML, Mullen B. A meta-analysis of the effect of oral and inhaled corticosteroids on growth. *J Allergy Clin Immunol* 1994;**93**:967–76.
4. Ilangovan P, Pedersen S, Godfrey S et al. Treatment of severe steroid dependent pre-school asthma with nebulised budesonide suspension. *Arch Dis Child* 1993;**68**:356–9.

15   Acute severe asthma

Parents and children need clear instructions about what to do when an acute asthma attack occurs and when to ask for medical help. If the attack does not respond quickly to the child's usual relief medication, treatment should be initiated at home with a large dose of a β_2-agonist bronchodilator. Up to 10 puffs salbutamol or terbutaline by MDI plus spacer (with or without a face mask) with one puff given every 15 to 30 seconds, or a nebulised bronchodilator therapy, is advised every three to four hours as an acceptable alternative while the family are seeking medical attention.

The response to treatment should be documented objectively in all children old enough to use a peak flow meter. A child who responds well to a high dose of bronchodilator at home will need to be reviewed a few hours later and will require increased prophylactic treatment (usually a doubling of inhaled steroid therapy) for a few weeks afterwards. Consideration should be given to starting a course of oral prednisolone at 1 to 2 mg/kg/day. If the child fails to respond, or relapses despite the above management, then commence oral prednisolone, give oxygen and arrange for transfer to hospital.

The principles of assessment and treatment in hospital of children over the age of 18 months are similar to those for adults, though some children recover without the need for systemic steroids. When faced with an intravenous infusion young children sometimes become extremely distressed, which can make their asthma worse, in which case it may be better to treat them with nebulised salbutamol, ipratropium bromide and a course of oral steroids.

Oxygen and dehydration
Oxygen is important in treatment but sometimes difficult to give to toddlers. They become dehydrated because of poor fluid intake, sweating and, in the early stages, hyperventilation. This must be corrected, but there are potential risks of overhydrating children with severe asthma. Production of antidiuretic hormone may be increased during the attack and the considerable negative intrathoracic pressures generated by the respiratory efforts may predispose to pulmonary oedema. After correcting dehydration the wisest course is to give normal fluid requirements and measure the plasma and urine osmolality.

Stabilisation
Children should not be discharged from hospital until they are taking the treatment that they will be taking at home and until their peak flow rate is at least 75% of expected or best known.

Indicators of acute severe asthma in children
- Child is too short of breath to talk or feed
- Respirations are >50 bpm (>40 bpm in >5 year olds)
- Pulse is >140 bpm (>120 bpm >5 year olds)
- Use of accessory muscles by child

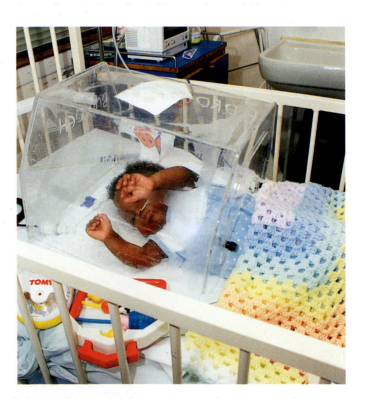

Infant requiring oxygen for management of acute severe asthma

Features of acute severe asthma

- Too breathless to talk or feed

- Respiratory rate
  >50 in under 5s
  >40 in over 5s

- Pulse rate
  >140 in under 5s
  >120 in over 5s

- Use of accessory muscles

- Peak flow <50% best or predicted
  (in over 5s)

Features of life threatening asthma

- Cyanosis, silent chest or poor respiratory effort

- Fatigue or exhaustion

- Agitation or reduced level of consciousness

- Peak flow <33% best or predicted (in over 5s)

Immediate treatment

- High flow oxygen via non-rebreathe mask to maintain SaO_2 >92%

- Nebulised β_2-agonist via oxygen driven nebuliser
  Salbutamol 2.5 mg in under 5s
  Salbutamol 5 mg in over 5s

- Prednisolone 1 to 2 mg/kg orally up to maximum 40 mg

- Consider iv access

If life-threatening features present

- Give iv salbutamol 4 to 6 micrograms per kilogram over 5 minutes, then 0.6 to 1 micrograms per kilogram per minute continuous infusion (this indication is unlicensed)
  or
  iv aminophylline 5 mg/kg over 20 minutes, then 900 micrograms per kilogram per hour continuous infusion;
  omit loading dose if child receiving aminophylline or theophylline

- iv hydrocortisone 4 to 8 mg/kg (max 200 mg) followed by doses of 2 to 4 mg/kg (max 100 mg) every six hours

- Add nebulised ipratropium 125 to 250 micrograms in under 5s; 250 to 500 micrograms in over 5s

- Consider chest X-ray if first episode of wheeze; SaO_2 <92%; or other clinical features indicate need

If child improving

- Continue as above

- Administer nebulised salbutamol every 1 to 4 hours

If no improvement within 15 to 30 minutes

- Increase salbutamol as needed, up to every 30 minutes or back to back

- Blood gases

- Transfer to ITU if increasing CO_2, decreasing O_2 exhaustion or respiratory arrest

Management of acute severe asthma in children

INDEX

Page numbers in **bold** refer to figures; those in *italic* refer to tables or boxed material

Accuhalers **43**, 44
acute asthma
    assessment 23
    examination 23–4
    features of 23
    treatment *25*, 26–31
    where to treat 24
acute severe asthma, children 62, *63*
adrenocorticotrophic hormone (ACTH) 39
adult height 12
aerosols 60
air pollution 49
air quality 21–2
airflow obstruction, recording 7
airways
    hyperresponsiveness 10
    inflammation 49
    nature of 2
allergens
    avoidance of 39–40
    in the home 17
allergic bronchopulmonary aspergillosis 18
Alternaria 18
alternative propellants 42–3
alternative therapies 40–1
aminophylline 20, 27
antibiotics 29
anticholinergic agents 27, 36
Aspergillus fumigatus 18
assessment
    acute asthma 23
    childhood asthma 53
asthma
    clinical course 12–15
    definition 1–2
    diagnostic testing and monitoring 7–11
    illness and diagnosis 50–3
    pathology 2–3
    precipitating factors 16–22
    prevalence 4–6
    types 3
    see also acute asthma; childhood asthma; chronic asthma
atenolol 20
atopic subjects 4
atopy 11, 46, *47*
Atropa belladonna **27**
Autohalers **37**, 43, 60

β-blockers 20
β-stimulants 26–7, 35
beclomethasone dipropionate 37–8
blood gases 24
breath actuated aerosol inhalers 43
breathlessness 23
British Thoracic Society (BTS) 14, 15, 55
bronchial hyperresponsiveness 16
bronchiolitis 50
bronchodilatation 35
bronchodilators
    anticholinergic 36
    childhood asthma 55–6
    combinations of 40
    response to 7–8
    use of 33
budesonide 37, 38

calcium antagonists 20
CFC-free inhalers 42–3
challenge tests 9
chest sounds 24
childhood asthma
    definition 45
    prevalence 45–6
    prevention 47–8
    reasons for increase in 46
    treatment 54–61
    trigger factors 48–9
    see also acute severe asthma
chronic asthma
    aims of management 33–4
    clinics 33
    general features 32–3
    guidelines 32
    treatment *34*, 35–41
chronic obstructive pulmonary disease (COPD) 2, 11, 26, 36
Cladosporium 18
Clickhalers 44
clinical course 12–15
clinical evidence 2–3
clinical histories 11
clinics 33
cockroaches 17
combined preparations 40
confidence 21
consultation, sympathetic 52

corticosteroids 28, 37–8, 39
cyclosporin 39

deadly nightshade **27**
deaths 13–14, 28
dehydration 62
Dermatophagoides pteronyssinus 17
desensitisation 39–40
diagnosis 52–3
diagnostic criteria 5
diagnostic testing 7–11
diary cards 7
diet 6
differential diagnosis 3, 11
discharge, from hospital 31
diurnal variation 8, 14
domestic environments 48
drug prophylaxis 16–17
drug treatment
    acute asthma 33–4
    childhood asthma 55–61
drug-induced asthma 20–1
drugs
    categories 14
    delivery 42–4
    pregnancy 22
dry powder inhalers 43–4, 60, 61
dust mites 17, 54

Easibreathe 43
education, patient 15, 42
eformoterol 35, 56
electrolytes 29
emotional factors 21
environment 6, 17, 48, 54
exercise 16–17
exercise testing 9
extension tubes **42**, 43
"extrinsic" asthma 3

family histories 5
fluids 29
fluticasone propionate 38
food allergy 19–20

general practice, acute asthma 25
genetics 4–5
"growing out", of asthma 12
growth, childhood 59
guidelines 32

height, adult 12
herbal preparations 41
histamine 10
home, allergens in 17, 54
hospitals
    discharge from 31
    treatment, acute asthma *30*
"hygiene hypothesis" 47
hypercapnia 24
hypersecretory asthma 52
hyposensitisation 18
hypoxia 24, 28

iatrogenic effects 20–1
ibuprofen 20
illness patterns 50–3
indoor environments 6
infections 6, 47
infusions 44
inhaled corticosteroids 37–8
inhaled steroids 57–9
inhalers 42–4, 57, 59, 60, 61
injections 44
"intrinsic" asthma 3
ionisation 41
ipratropium bromide 20, 27, 36

labelling 1–2, 53
leukotriene antagonists 9, 39, 44
leukotriene receptor antagonists 33, 56
long acting β-agonists 35–6
long acting β2–agonists 56
lung function tests 52
lymphocytes 47

management
    acute asthma 31
    childhood asthma *58*
    chronic asthma 33–4
    partnerships 54
management plans **7**, 15
mast cell stabilisers 37
maternal smoking 5, *47*
mechanical ventilation 29
metered dose inhalers (MDI) 42, 43, 57
methacholine responsiveness 5
methotrexate 39
methylxanthines 27–8, 36–7
metoprolol 20
mild asthma 53
moderate asthma 53
monitoring 7–11
montelukast 56
morbidity 15
mortality 13–15, 28
mucus plugging 3

nebulisers 26–7, 29, 44, 55–6, 60–1
nedocromil sodium 37
New Zealand, mortality 13–14
nitrogen dioxide 22
nocturnal attacks 9
non-asthmatic wheezing 11
non-specific stimuli 16

occupational asthma 19
Odense Study 5
older patients 2
oral agents 59
oral corticosteroids 39
outdoor tests 9
oxitropium bromide 36
oxygen 28–9, 62

parenteral delivery 27
pathology 2–3

patients
  education 15, 42
  inhaler preferences 61
peak expiratory flow rate (PEFR) 56
peak flow meters **2**, 7, 15
peak flow monitoring 23, 24
peak flow variation 8–9
pets 18
pollens 18, 40
pollution 21–2, 49
potassium supplements 29
powders 60
precipitating factors 16–22
predictability 50–1
prednisolone 28, 39, 55
pregnancy 5, 22
presentation 52
prevalence 4–6, 45–7
prognosis, adults 12–13
prophylactic agents 56
prophylaxis 2
prostaglandin synthetase inhibitors 20
public health issues 46
Pulsus paradoxus 24

rapid response 14
refractoriness 17
relaxation 21, 41
remission 12
rescue intervention 55
respiratory tract infections 50
reversibility 7–8
Rotahalers 60

salicyclates 20
salmeterol 35, 56
seasonal asthma 53

self management plans **7**, 54
severe asthma 53
skin tests 10–11
smoking 5, 6, *47*, 48
sodium cromoglycate 20, 37, 57
specific airway challenge 10
spores 18
stabilisation 62
steroid sparing agents 39
steroids 28, 37–8, 39, 57–9
symptoms, childhood asthma 45
syrups 44

T lymphocytes 47
tablets 44
teenagers 51–2
Th2 cells 2, 47
theophylline 27, 28, 33, 36–7, 44, 59
treatment plans 7
Turbohalers 44, 60

United Kingdom, mortality 13

ventilation, controlled 29–30
vocal cord dysfunction 11
volume spacers 26, **37**, 38, 56, 60, 61

weather 22
weight control 5
wheezing
  drug regime 33
  infants 1, 50, 52
  non-asthmatic 11
  prevalence *4*, 5

zafirlukast 39, 56
zileuton 39